Good Cholesterol, Bad Cholesterol

Eli M. Roth, M.D., F.A.C.C.

Sandra L. Streicher-Lankin, R.N.

PRIMA HEALTH

A Division of Prima Publishing

For Dan, my husband, friend, love, and inspiration. Thank you for your constant loving support. Since living with you, I know the most important element to keeping a heart healthy—love.

Sandy

Library of Congress Cataloging-in-Publication Data

Roth, Eli.
    Good cholesterol, bad cholesterol / Eli M. Roth and Sandra L. Streicher-Lankin.—Rev. and updated 2nd ed.
      p.   cm.
    Includes index.
    ISBN 0-7615-0010-3
    1. Coronary heart disease—Prevention—Popular works.
2. Atherosclerosis—Prevention—Popular works. 3. Hypercholesterolemia—Prevention—Popular works. 4. Blood Cholesterol—Popular works. 5. Low-cholesterol diet—Popular works.
I. Streicher-Lankin, Sandra L. II. Title.
RC685.C6R686 1995
616.1'2305—dc20
                                            95-5285
                                          CIP

99 AA 9 8 7 6 5 4

Printed in the United States of America

The HEARTSMART™ Program referred to in this book was copyrighted in 1986 by Eli M. Roth, M.D., and Sandra L. Streicher-Lankin, R.N. The name HEARTSMART™ is a registered trademark in the state of Ohio and is not associated in any way with any product or program bearing a similar name.

How to Order:

Single copies may be ordered from Prima Publishing, P.O. Box 1260BK, Rocklin, CA 95677; telephone (916) 632-4400. Quantity discounts are also available. On your letterhead, include information concerning the intended use of the books and the number of books you wish to purchase.

Contents

Foreword

Coronary artery disease today remains the number one cause of death in the United States.

The public seems infatuated with spectacular cases of the total artificial heart and transplantation in dealing with endstage coronary artery disease. However, seemingly as unpopular as it may appear, the much more effective means of combatting coronary artery disease is in the prevention of the disease by the adaptation of lifestyle.

Good Cholesterol, Bad Cholesterol provides a comprehensive source of information on cholesterol in an easily understood fashion. The book explains the physiological impact of cholesterol and the significance of its management and control. The authors furnish an account of different types of lipids in the blood and types of dietary fats. There is an informative chapter on label reading and an explanation of how the blood lipid levels are tested, as well as the current National Institutes of Health and American Heart Association recommendations.

This book provides a general overview of how to obtain and maintain recommended lipid levels and discusses the different medications used to treat lipid disorders not manageable with dietary alterations only. The reader is afforded with practical information on hints for dining out in restaurants and some recipe ideas.

I believe this book offers the general public a valuable insight into the benefits of a disease preventative lifestyle.

William C. DeVries, M.D.

Preface

There is now no question that cholesterol is linked to heart disease. Multiple studies have shown a direct relationship between abnormal cholesterol levels and increased risk of heart disease. More important, several studies in recent years have shown that decreasing cholesterol levels do result in a lower incidence of heart attack. It is for this reason that the public has been bombarded with cholesterol information. As a cardiologist and cardiovascular nurse, we are all too familiar with the result of elevated cholesterol—heart attack, stroke, and weakening and blockages in other arteries (atherosclerosis). Our patients have asked for easy to read, understandable information about cholesterol. They wanted something other than a list of "Do's and Don'ts" and needed information and advice that could be used for a lifetime—not a temporary "fad diet." We searched for this type of information, and were unable to find it in any one source. There is a great deal of cholesterol information available, but we feel this book is the first to bring it all together in a readable, easy to understand, medically correct form. This book gives accurate information and provides basic behavior modification principles which make lifetime eating habit changes possible. *Good Cholesterol, Bad Cholesterol* will not only explain what to do, but it will help you to understand why. A great deal of time and effort went into the research and writing of this book. We feel that the end result reflects our efforts and that the book does fulfill the goals which we set.

We want to extend heartfelt thanks to Steven Martin, developmental editor, and Betsy Towner, assistant project editor, at Prima Publishing for their invaluable assistance. Their editorial acumen helped in improving this manuscript and getting it to publication. It was both a pleasure and a professionally enriching experience working with both of them.

EMR and SLSL

1   Why Worry about Cholesterol?

Why should anyone worry about something they really can't see, let alone understand? According to the American Heart Association, 1.5 million people will suffer a heart attack in the coming year, and of those, more than 500,000 people will die. Heart attacks are caused by coronary heart disease, also known as coronary artery disease (blockages in the blood vessels supplying blood to the heart). Elevated blood cholesterol is a major cause of these blockages. In addition, these blockages (also known as atherosclerosis) can and do form in any of the arteries in the body. This can lead to stroke, high blood pressure, blood supply problems to the legs, or an aneurysm (a weak spot or bulging in the arteries).

Fortunately, by controlling the blood cholesterol level, formation of these blockages can be slowed or even stopped. Over the past eighty years, many research studies have clearly proven that elevated blood cholesterol levels cause an increase in atherosclerosis and coronary artery disease. Then why has the fuss over cholesterol just occurred in the last ten years? Because, until 1984, no study proved that lowering the blood cholesterol levels would reduce the risk of developing coronary artery disease and heart attacks. Then in 1984, Lipid Research Clinics Coronary Primary Prevention Trial (LRC CPPT) proved without a doubt that lowering cholesterol levels did lower the risk of heart attack. This study, conducted by the National Institutes of Health, is considered the cornerstone study on cholesterol. The study, conducted in twelve centers in North America, involved 3,806 men*, took ten years to complete, and cost $150 million. The LRC CPPT established that lowering the blood cholesterol does lower the risk of suffering a fatal or nonfatal heart attack.

The results of ten years of follow-up in these men demonstrated that for every 1% the blood cholesterol is lowered, the risk of heart attack is lowered 2%! In other words, two groups of men—identical as far as age, weight, smoking, blood pressure, etc.—were compared to each other. These groups, which stayed identical other than cholesterol level, had a marked difference in the occurrence of heart attack. For example, a man in the cholesterol-controlled group who lowered his cholesterol blood level 10% had a 20% less chance of a heart attack than if he had not lowered his cholesterol. Since the LRC CPPT, dozens of large, well-planned studies have shown similar and consistent results: lowering cholesterol decreases atherosclerosis (blockages in the arteries) and heart attack risk.

*The National Institutes of Health Consensus Development Conference Statement on Lowering Blood Cholesterol to Prevent Heart Disease states: "This benefit of lowering cholesterol has been demonstrated most conclusively in men with elevated blood cholesterol levels, but much evidence justifies the conclusion that similar protection will be afforded to women with elevated levels."

So what are you waiting for? Reduce your blood cholesterol level and reduce your chance of heart disease. Since most of the cholesterol in the blood comes from food containing cholesterol or saturated fats, learning how to control and modify your eating is the first step to lower cholesterol. This book will teach you to understand and conquer cholesterol. You will learn what your recommended cholesterol level should be, how to have the cholesterol level in the blood properly checked, and what medications your physician can prescribe to help lower the cholesterol level if proper diet alone is not sufficient. Most importantly, when you finish this book you will understand cholesterol enough to make dietary management easier, as well as practical and palatable. You will learn how to eat as if your life depends on it.

CHOLESTEROL AND CARDIOVASCULAR DISEASE

Cholesterol is a major contributing cause of cardiovascular disease. Cardiovascular disease is a general term used to describe problems with the blood vessels or heart. Approximately 70 million Americans have some form of cardiovascular disease. Atherosclerosis, the most common form, is a progressive condition that affects the arteries or "tubes" that carry blood, oxygen, and nutrients to the body as well as to the heart itself. As the heart pumps, or beats, it moves the blood through these tubes. Normally, the inside of the arteries are smooth, and they expand and contract with each heartbeat as the blood flows through them. But in atherosclerosis there is a buildup of cholesterol, fat, and calcium within the smooth inside lining of the artery. This buildup gradually becomes hardened. For this reason atherosclerosis is frequently called hardening of the arteries. Not only does atherosclerosis cause the inside of the artery to narrow so that less blood can flow through, it also decreases the ability of the artery to expand and contract.

The arteries that supply the heart with blood are called the coronary arteries. When the coronary arteries are affected by atherosclerosis, the heart does not receive the blood supply it needs, and the result could be a heart attack. The development of atherosclerosis is dependent upon the buildup of cholesterol, fats, and other substances within the arteries. Therefore, if you reduce the amount of cholesterol and fats in the blood, you will decrease the development and progression of atherosclerosis. The best way to begin to reduce your blood cholesterol level is to limit the amount of cholesterol in your diet and modify the kinds of fats you eat.

2   Lipids and Cholesterol

People use so many different terms when talking about cholesterol that it can become confusing. Before we start with how to control your cholesterol, let's get a better understanding of these terms and the language of cholesterol.

What are lipids? Lipids are fats. Lipid is the most general term used to describe all the fats within the body. The body needs certain amounts and kinds of fats to function properly. Just as oil and water do not mix, lipids (oil) and blood (water) will not mix. For lipids to be transported in the bloodstream and put to use in the body, they combine with proteins. These lipid-protein combinations are called lipoproteins. Since fats combine with proteins to do the work that is required of them, the terms lipid and lipoprotein mean the same thing for all practical purposes.

The general category of lipids is made up of several different kinds of fats. As you will see and understand, some lipids cause the development and progression of atherosclerosis, while other lipids are actually helpful in preventing atherosclerosis.

One category of blood lipids is cholesterol. Our understanding of cholesterol, and specifically the different types of cholesterol, has increased tremendously over the past several years. Cholesterol can be divided into two major types. The first type is the Low Density Lipoprotein cholesterol. It is known as *LDL cholesterol*. LDL is the bad cholesterol. LDL cholesterol is the fat that enters the inside lining of the artery and causes atherosclerosis. The second type of cholesterol is the High Density Lipoprotein cholesterol. This is known as *HDL cholesterol*. HDL is the good cholesterol. This particular kind of cholesterol actually fights against atherosclerosis and the buildup of fat in the arteries. There are other types of cholesterol, but the two major groups are LDL and HDL.

Another group of blood lipids is known as triglycerides. Triglycerides are one of the lipids that we know the least about. However, research has shown that elevated triglyceride levels are correlated with an increased incidence of atherosclerosis (see Chapter 3). In general, LDL cholesterol appears to be a much more important factor in the development of atherosclerosis than triglycerides.

To review, the term lipid or lipoprotein refers to any fat in the body. The primary kinds of lipids in the blood are cholesterol and triglycerides. Within the category of cholesterol, we have two major types: the bad cholesterol known as LDL and the good cholesterol known as HDL.

WHERE DOES CHOLESTEROL COME FROM?

Cholesterol is actually an important substance that many different body tissues and hormones use to function. Because of its importance, your body has the ability to produce, or synthesize, cholesterol. Cholesterol that is produced by the body is said to be "endogenous." All animals (as well as fish and fowl) produce and utilize cholesterol within their bodies. The majority of cholesterol in your body, however, actually comes from eating (ingesting) foods that contain cholesterol and saturated fat. This will be explained further in Chapter 4. These foods are mainly of animal origin. Cholesterol that is obtained from outside sources is termed "exogenous."

The total amount of cholesterol the body requires is relatively small. Therefore, the majority of the cholesterol within the bloodstream is more than the body needs. It is this excess cholesterol that enters the walls of the arteries and forms deposits (or plaques), the beginning of atherosclerosis and, more specifically, coronary artery disease in the heart. Since the majority of the cholesterol within the bloodstream is from exogenous sources, limiting cholesterol and saturated fat intake will normally have a significant effect on lowering blood cholesterol levels. *The lowering of blood cholesterol levels has been shown to slow the progression of atherosclerosis and coronary artery disease.*

NORMAL LEVELS VERSUS RECOMMENDED LEVELS

In the last decade, we have learned that there is a definite difference between the "normal" and "recommended" levels of cholesterol in the blood. The levels of cholesterol that have been considered "normal" for a long time are actually too high and are above the current "recommended" blood cholesterol levels. Simply stated, the American public has had high cholesterol for quite some time. These high levels are almost always the result of the usual American diet, which is high in cholesterol and saturated fats. The blood cholesterol levels that were considered normal in the past are really an average (or mean) of blood cholesterol levels found in a wide cross-section of people. These levels were never correlated with the occurrence of atherosclerosis or coronary artery disease until recently. The "recommended" levels are based on the levels of risk of developing coronary artery disease. The "Desirable Blood Cholesterol" level is less than 200 mg/dL (milligrams per deciliter). Cholesterol levels of 200–239 mg/dL are considered "Borderline-High Blood Cholesterol" and greater than 240 mg/dL is considered "High Blood Cholesterol." If the blood cholesterol level is within the borderline-high range, then dietary changes should be made to lower the cholesterol level. When the level is at or above the high-risk level, diet modification is attempted first. If diet alone is not successful, medication to lower cholesterol should be used in combination with dietary changes. In general, the lower the blood cholesterol level, the less the chance of development of coronary artery disease. More detailed information about the recommended levels will be given in Chapter 7.

BLOOD CHOLESTEROL LEVELS	
Less than 200 mg/dL	Desirable
200–239 mg/dL	Borderline-high
Greater than or equal to 240 mg/dL	High

3 Triglycerides

Triglycerides are one of the lipids in the blood. Triglycerides function as a very efficient energy storage unit for the body. Their importance as a fuel can be seen from the fact that a person could fast for several weeks and survive by metabolizing their triglycerides for energy. In contrast, carbohydrates (sugars) are stored in amounts sufficient to last only a few hours.

Triglycerides can get into the bloodstream and tissues by two different routes. Dietary fats are transported from the intestine into the bloodstream, and then are usually stored in adipose (fat) cells for later use. If dietary fat is replaced with carbohydrates, then the liver will make the sugars into triglycerides. This is done by special chemicals (enzymes) within the liver. The triglycerides are then secreted into the blood and removed by fat cells just the same as dietary triglycerides. The purpose for the conversion of carbohydrates to triglycerides is because the lipids are much better energy storage units. A gram of fat has nine calories whereas a gram of carbohydrates has four calories. In addition to triglycerides having more than twice the calories of carbohydrates, lipids have many more storage sites (fat cells) than sugars do.

When they are needed for energy, triglycerides are broken down into free fatty acids and glycerol in the fat cells. Several physiologic conditions cause this release to occur. These include physical activity, fasting, stress, and uncontrolled diabetes. The free fatty acids and glycerol are then transported in the blood from the fat cells to the site at which the energy is needed (for example, in the leg muscles when one jogs for several miles).

LIPID METABOLISM AND RESEARCH

Triglycerides are an important part of lipid metabolism or use of lipids within the body. It is important to realize that the concepts presented in this book have been simplified, so as to help better explain the ideas of blood lipids, dietary fats, and atherosclerosis. It is also important to realize that lipid research is an ongoing process. We understand only a fraction of everything there is to know about lipids. Of all the lipids, triglycerides are the least studied and understood. Because of this, the information about triglycerides is limited. Presented below sums up what we think we presently understand about triglycerides and their role in atherosclerosis.

ATHEROSCLEROTIC RISK

In general, triglycerides are thought to cause less atherosclerosis than other lipids such as LDL cholesterol. Multiple studies have suggested that coronary heart disease does not correspond to triglyceride levels. However, limited other studies disagree with this.

It is generally thought that triglycerides are an independent risk factor for atherosclerosis in women but not in men. There is an inverse relationship between blood triglyceride levels and HDL cholesterol levels that tends to confuse this issue. This means that when the fasting triglyceride levels tend to be increased, the HDL (good) cholesterol levels tend to be lower than normal. As you have learned, HDL (good) cholesterol protects against atherosclerosis and coronary heart disease. Therefore, an elevated triglyceride level (and thus decreased HDL cholesterol level) may cause atherosclerosis indirectly.

Most of the large cholesterol studies mentioned earlier in the book focused on either total cholesterol or LDL cholesterol levels and atherosclerosis. When two groups—one taking medication and the other not—were compared, the medications were aimed at lowering LDL and total cholesterol. There have really been no large studies specifically designed to look at the effect of lowering triglycerides. (In the same way, there have been no studies completed to date specifically designed to look at the effect of raising HDL cholesterol levels.)

It is important to realize that triglycerides, LDL cholesterol, and HDL cholesterol are all interrelated. The formation of all these different lipids is a result of a common process which links one to another. Therefore, it is difficult to change the blood level of one of these lipids with medication without having some effect on the others. This makes it difficult to get a "pure effect" of the medication.

HIGH TRIGLYCERIDE LEVELS

There are several situations in which high triglyceride levels are commonly seen. These include diabetes, obesity, high calorie intake in an overweight individual, alcohol consumption, a high-carbohydrate diet, and a sedentary lifestyle. Steps can be taken to decrease the blood triglyceride levels without the use of medications. Obviously, weight loss and exercise would be very beneficial to decreasing triglyceride levels. Good glucose control in diabetes by diet, exercise, and oral medication and/or insulin is also beneficial. Decreasing or stopping alcohol consumption will help lower triglyceride levels as well as reduce calorie intake. A high carbohydrate diet can lead to increased triglyceride levels and should not be done without professional guidance.

Triglyceride levels can be quite elevated in a non-fasting state, especially immediately after a meal. It is therefore important to test blood triglyceride levels in an adequately fasted state. All recommendations concerning triglyceride blood levels are based on a fasting state (twelve hours without food intake).

ABNORMAL BLOOD LEVELS

Triglyceride levels above 500 mg/dL are considered high and between 250–500 mg/dL are considered borderline-high. Elevated triglyceride levels should always be treated by lifestyle changes before medications are considered. However, extremely high triglyceride levels and triglyceride levels refractory to lifestyle changes should be treated with medications. More information on this can be found in Chapter 13.

4 Understanding Fats in Food

Various types of fats are found in many of the foods you eat, and your body uses these fats in totally different ways. The three basic categories of dietary fats found in food are cholesterol, "saturated fats," and "unsaturated fats." Unsaturated fats can be further divided into "monounsaturated" and "polyunsaturated." Eating cholesterol-rich foods will obviously increase your blood cholesterol level. Ingesting saturated fats also raises your blood cholesterol level, whereas unsaturated fats will actually lower your cholesterol level. For this reason it is important for you to understand and recognize each category. Information on cholesterol in foods as well as cholesterol dietary recommendations will be covered in Chapter 5. The remainder of this chapter will deal with saturated and unsaturated fats.

Saturated fats raise the blood cholesterol level, which in turn causes the development and progression of atherosclerosis. Therefore, you want to limit the intake of saturated fats in your diet. How can you tell if a product contains saturated fat? Examining the product label will tell what kind of fats are contained in the food (see Chapter 6). Foods are now labeled with not only the total fat content, but also the saturated fat content in grams and the percent of calories from fat. If the label does not tell you the saturated fat content, there are two rules of thumb you can follow to determine if saturated fats are present. The first rule is that saturated fats are solid at room temperature. The second rule is that dairy products and any food made from animal sources are high in saturated fats. (This may make more sense if you remember that milk comes from an animal source.) The only two exceptions to these rules are palm and coconut oils. Although they are from vegetable sources and can be in liquid form, both are high in saturated fat.

To help reduce the amount of saturated fat in your diet, you must avoid or limit foods that are high in saturated fats. This would include solid shortenings, fatty meats, products made from animal fat, and dairy products. Butter, cream, and whole milk contain cholesterol as well as saturated fats. Therefore, anything made from these dairy products contains both saturated fat and cholesterol. Some examples of this are ice cream, cheese, and baked goods. The saturated fat content of dairy products can be lowered. Whole milk contains 3.5% butterfat. The lower butterfat content is signified by a percent in the labeling, such as 2%, 1%, or .5%. The American Heart Association recommends the use of .5% milk (skim milk is .5% or lower) for all adults and children over two years of age.

In summary, saturated fats are one type of fat found in the foods you eat. Saturated fats raise the cholesterol level in the blood and should be limited in your diet. Saturated fats are usually solid at room temperature and are found in foods from animal sources and dairy products. Palm and coconut oils are also high in saturated fat and should be avoided.

Let's see how the two rules of thumb about saturated fats can help you decide if a product is a wise low-fat choice.

Is lard a saturated fat? The answer is yes. It is a solid fat at room temperature, and it is made from animal products. Both rules of determining saturated fats apply to lard.

Does whole milk contain saturated fat? Yes, whole milk is a dairy product so, according to the second rule, it does contain saturated fat. Whole milk has a high butterfat (saturated fat) content.

Is liquid corn oil high in saturated fat? No. Corn oil is liquid at room temperature and is made from vegetable as opposed to animal sources. (It does not contain the exceptions of palm or coconut oil.)

Does "all vegetable shortening" contain saturated fat? The answer is yes. Although the shortening is made from vegetable sources, it is a solid at room temperature. The first rule tells you it is a saturated fat. Generally, the term "shortening" refers to a solid form whereas "oil" refers to a liquid form. Many solid vegetable products are advertised as "Cholesterol Free" or "Contains No Cholesterol." These statements are true. They do not contain cholesterol, but they do contain saturated fat, which raises the cholesterol level in your blood. That is why it is so important for you to understand all of the factors that go into controlling your cholesterol.

Does "nondairy coffee creamer" contain saturated fat? The answer is maybe. Some nondairy creamers contain palm or coconut oil, both of which contain saturated fats. If you add creamer to your coffee, the best choice would be either a nondairy coffee creamer without palm or coconut oil, or skim milk.

WHAT ARE POLYUNSATURATED FATS?

Another type of fat found in the foods you eat is called polyunsaturated. The polyunsaturated fats tend to lower the cholesterol level in the blood. They do this by enabling the body to eliminate newly formed cholesterol that is excessive. Polyunsaturates are found in fish oils and liquid oils made from vegetables. Once again, the exceptions to this are palm and coconut oils.

Polyunsaturated fats can be changed to become solid at room temperature. This process is known as hydrogenation and forms what is called a "trans" fatty acid. When a polyunsaturated fat has been hydrogenated, it behaves like a saturated fat in the body and causes an increase in the blood cholesterol level. Foods may either be partially or completely hydrogenated. Many of the liquid vegetable oils are partially hydrogenated to produce margarine and other products. Foods containing oil that has been partially hydrogenated may be an acceptable low-fat food. In general, hydrogenated oils should be considered as saturated fats, whereas partially hydrogenated oils are considered polyunsaturates. The softer the hydrogenated oil is, the less saturated it has become.

The way to identify a good low-fat food choice is to read the label. If the food contains a minimum of twice as much polyunsaturated as saturated fat, it is considered acceptable. Saturated fats raise the blood cholesterol level twice as much as an equal amount of polyunsaturated fat lowers the blood cholesterol level. By following the 2:1 ratio of polyunsaturated:

saturated, the blood cholesterol level will remain unchanged. By consuming more polyunsaturates than this, the blood cholesterol level can actually be lowered.

EXAMPLES OF POLYUNSATURATED VEGETABLE FATS	
Corn oil	Soybean oil
Sunflower oil	Cottonseed oil
Safflower oil	Liquid all-vegetable oil

Fish Oil Polyunsaturated Fats

Under the category of unsaturated fats are the vegetable polyunsaturates, which we have just discussed, and fish oils. For many years little attention was paid to polyunsaturated fish oils. Then in the 1970s, a very important study examined the rarity of heart disease among the Eskimos in Greenland. This study found that their diet was limited almost exclusively to fish and fish products. It was interesting to the researchers that people who ate oily fish had virtually no heart disease. Because of this observation, fish oils were closely examined. Scientists have discovered that the polyunsaturates found in some cold-water, deep-sea fish are very effective in lowering blood cholesterol. It is now recognized that these polyunsaturates will lower blood cholesterol levels more than an equal amount of vegetable polyunsaturates, but it is difficult to ingest enough fish oils in food to lower the cholesterol level significantly. For this reason, companies are manufacturing fish oils in capsule or gelatin form that can be taken as a dietary supplement.

Vegetable and Fish Oil Polyunsaturates

About now you're probably asking yourself, "What's the difference between vegetable polyunsaturates and fish oil polyunsaturates if they both lower the blood cholesterol level?" That's a good question. The primary differences are in the chemical structure and in the way the body utilizes the fat, based on that chemical structure. Fats are made up of complex chains of fatty acids that occur naturally. In most unsaturated fats, the first double bond (the unsaturated area) occurs in a certain position along the fatty acid chain. This position is called omega-6. Vegetable polyunsaturates are desaturated in this omega-6 position. However, fish oils are desaturated in a different area, the omega-3 position. This simple difference of desaturation position appears to make a major difference in the cholesterol-lowering ability of the fish oil polyunsaturates compared to the vegetable polyunsaturates. In addition, the fish oils are longer in length and generally more unsaturated than the vegetable oils. Fish oils are especially rich in a long-chain omega-3 fatty acid known as EPA (eicosapentaenoic acid). We mention all of these names because the manufacturers of fish oil supplements are using these terms to make up names for their products. Some examples of these names are ProMega, ProtoChol, Cardi-Omega 3, and MaxEPA.

Again, the body's use of any substance is dependent upon that substance's chemical structure. In this case, the omega-3 position appears to be a more potent agent for reducing blood cholesterol than the omega-6 position. The longer length of the omega-3 fatty acid chain and the increased number of desaturated areas within the chain (double bonds) may also be important factors in the fish oils' ability to lower cholesterol.

Interestingly, the fish and fish oils that are high in omega-3 polyunsaturates are also high in cholesterol. As you have just learned, ingesting cholesterol will raise your blood cholesterol level. Despite this high cholesterol content, the omega-3 polyunsaturates still cause an overall lowering of the blood cholesterol level. This suggests that they are a potent cholesterol-lowering agent. In addition, several of the fish oil supplements are now cholesterol-free due to special processing. If fish oil supplements are used, these cholesterol-free supplements are recommended. There is still controversy as to the benefit of fish oil and fish oil supplements in lowering cholesterol. We recommend that you consult with your physician if you are considering the use of fish oil supplements. Remember that polyunsaturated fats from any source lower total blood cholesterol.

In Table 4.1 we have listed some foods that are high in omega-3 fatty acids. Notice the high cholesterol content of the fish sources.

ALL POLYUNSATURATED FATS AND OILS ARE NOT CREATED EQUAL

All of the oils and fats that you eat contain saturated, polyunsaturated, and monounsaturated fats. Monounsaturated fats are a special type of polyunsaturate. They contain only one (mono) double bond, instead of many (poly) double bonds found in the polyunsaturated fats. Previously it was believed that monounsaturated fats did not lower or raise the blood cholesterol level. More recently, several studies have shown that monounsaturates do indeed lower the blood cholesterol level. In fact, monounsaturates lower the LDL (bad) cholesterol level without affecting the

Table 4.1   Sources of Omega-3 Fatty Acids in Foods
(per 100 grams raw edible portion)

Food	Omega-3 Fatty Acids (g)	Cholesterol (g)
Cod liver oil	19.2	570
Salmon oil	20.9	485
Bass (fresh water)	0.3	59
Cod (Atlantic)	0.3	43
Halibut (Pacific)	0.5	32
Mackerel (Atlantic)	2.6	80
Perch (white)	0.4	80
Salmon (pink)	1.0	—*
Tuna (albacore)	1.5	54
Trout (lake)	2.0	48
Crab (Alaska king)	0.3	—
Shrimp (Atlantic)	0.3	142
Clam (soft shell)	0.4	—
Walnut oil	10.4	0
Butternuts (dried)	8.7	0
Soybean oil	6.8	0
Walnuts (black)	3.3	0
Beans (common, dry)	0.6	0
Strawberries	0.1	0

*A dash indicates the lack of data available for nutrient known to be present.

Adapted from F. N. Hepburn and others, *Journal of the American Dietetic Association*

HDL (good) cholesterol level. These same studies suggest that polyunsaturates lower the blood cholesterol level by lowering both LDL and HDL cholesterol levels. Because of this, it is more prudent to substitute monounsaturates for polyunsaturates in your diet. Saturated fats elevate your total cholesterol, principally by elevating the LDL cholesterol. Polyunsaturated and monounsaturated fats lower your total cholesterol. For this reason you will want to choose oils that have the

Table 4.2

Type of Fat	Percent Polyunsaturated	Percent Saturated
Safflower oil	74%	9%
Sunflower oil	64%	10%
Corn oil	58%	13%
Vegetable oil (soybean and cottonseed)	40%	13%
Peanut oil	30%	19%
Chicken fat (schmaltz)	26%	29%
Olive oil	9%	14%
Vegetable Shortening	20%	32%
Lard	12%	40%
Beef Fat	4%	48%
Butter	4%	61%
Palm oil	2%	81%
Coconut oil	2%	86%

highest percentage of unsaturated fat, mono or poly (see Tables 4.2 and 4.3). In addition, monounsaturates are the preferred unsaturated fat because they lower LDL and not HDL cholesterol. Since all fats and oils contain 9 calories/gram (see Chapter 5), caloric intake will not be a factor in the type of oil you choose.

Table 4.3

Type of Oil	Percent Polyunsaturated	Percent Monounsaturated	Percent Saturated
Olive oil	9%	77%	14%
Peanut oil	30%	51%	19%
Safflower oil	74%	17%	9%
Sunflower oil	64%	26%	10%
Corn oil	58%	29%	13%
Canola oil	29%	58%	7%

5 Your Daily Intake of Cholesterol and Fats

An apple a day may not keep the doctor away, but the American Heart Association, the National Cholesterol Education Program of the National Institutes of Health, and numerous medical professionals (including these authors) agree that a nutritious low-fat diet will help keep heart disease away. In previous chapters we have helped you understand and identify the different types of dietary fat. In this chapter we will put that knowledge into practical everyday use. Specific guidelines will be given and explained. In addition, examples and samples are provided to help you use this information in your daily eating plan. The following recommendations follow the guidelines set out by the American Heart Association and the National Institutes of Health. These guidelines are recommended for all Americans over the age of two:

- The total intake of dietary fats should be reduced to 30% or less of the total daily calories.

- The 30% or less of calories from fat should be divided as follows:

8–10% from saturated fat

up to 15% from monounsaturated fats

about 7%, not to exceed 10%, from polyunsaturated fats

- Reduce the dietary intake of cholesterol to 200–300 mg a day or less.
- Total daily calorie intake should be reduced to correct obesity and maintain ideal body weight and composition.

The dietary restrictions as listed above constitute what is referred to as the Step I diet. The Step I diet is recommended for all Americans over the age of two and is consistent with good nutrition. The Step I diet is the first step on the way to controlling cholesterol. If a Step I diet fails to control the blood cholesterol and bring it into an acceptable range, further dietary restrictions may be achieved by advancing to the Step II diet. The Step II diet is to be followed on the advice of your physician and should include counseling by a professional qualified to provide nutritional advice.

Since the Step I diet is the recommendation for the general public, we will be examining how to incorporate the Step I diet into your daily eating plan. If you must progress to the Step II diet on the recommendation of your physician, you will continue to apply the same principles and guidelines described in this book, but with stricter limitations.

In order to apply these recommendations, there are some facts you need to know and some calculations you will need to make. First you must know (or calculate) your average daily intake of calories. The daily intake of calories by Americans varies widely. It is essential that you keep track of your calorie intake for several days so that you can establish your specific average daily calorie intake. The average intake for women is about 1,800 calories a day, for men about 2,500 calories a day.

The second fact that you must know to calculate your daily fat calorie intake is that one gram of fat provides 9 calories. This is a universal, scientific truth and does *not* change dependent on whether or not the fat is saturated or unsaturated. All fats, regardless of saturation, contribute 9 calories per gram. For your additional information, one gram of protein provides 4 calories, as does one gram of carbohydrate. You can see that, gram for gram, fat contains more than twice as many calories as does protein and carbohydrate. For this reason, if you just shift your fat intake from saturated to unsaturated fats, either monounsaturated or polyunsaturated, your caloric intake will not change. If your caloric intake remains stable, without an increase in activity, you will not see a reduction in your weight. Remember that controlling your weight was one goal of the Step I diet.

Once you know your average daily calorie intake, you can calculate your 30% or less allowable calorie intake from fat by multiplying by .30. For example, if your daily calorie intake was 1,800 calories, your allowable calorie intake from fat would be no more than 30% of 1,800 (.30 × 1,800) or 540 calories. To find the number of grams that 540 calories of allowable fat intake is equal to, you would divide 540 by 9 since each gram of fat contains 9 calories. This would tell us that our total daily intake of fat on an 1,800 calorie diet is 60 grams of fat.

Let's take this same example one step further. Remember that the recommendation states that the total fat calorie intake is restricted in its composition. We have completed the first phase of the calculations by limiting the total fat intake to 30% or less. It is now necessary to break down that 30% into saturated, monounsaturated, and polyunsaturated fats. Next we will calculate the grams of saturated fat using the same 1,800 calorie diet. The saturated fat intake should be between 8–10% of the total fat calories. We know that the total fat for this 1,800-calorie diet is 540 calories or 60 grams. We must take 10% of the 1,800 calories (.10 × 1,800). No more than 180 of our calories can come from saturated fats. To determine how many grams of fat that equals, we would divide by 9 once again (180/9). Our allowable saturated fat intake would be 20 grams.

Now let's calculate the monounsaturated fats. Up to 15% of the total fat intake may be from mono-unsaturated fats (.15 × 1,800), and 15% of the 1,800 calories is 270 calories. Once again we will divide the calories by 9 to give us the grams of fat (270/9). We can eat 30 grams of monounsaturated fat on our 1,800-calorie diet.

To complete the picture, we have the polyunsatu-rated fats in our 1,800-calorie diet to calculate. Polyun-saturated fats should be about 7% of the total fat intake but must not exceed 10%. We will use the 7% for our calculations since we have already done a 10% calcu-lation (the saturated fat allowance above), and .07 × 1,800 equals 126. This means 126 calories can come from polyunsaturated fat. To find how many fat grams that is equal to, we will divide 126 by 9 (126/9). That means 14 grams of polyunsaturated fat can be eaten in an 1,800 calorie diet.

By doing these calculations, it's easy to put a Step I diet to work for you following the recommen-dations. These calculations combined with label read-ing can help you gain control of your cholesterol. To illustrate how the Step I diet recommendations work with various calorie ranges, we have included Table

Table 5.1 Maximum Daily Intake of Fat, Saturated Fat, and Cholesterol

Total Daily Calorie Intake	1,600	1,800	2,000	2,200	2,400	2,600	2,800	3,000
Total grams of fat	53	60	67	73	80	87	93	100
Grams of saturated fat	18	20	22	24	27	29	31	33
Cholesterol (in mg)	300	300	300	300	300	300	300	300

5.1. Next we list seven steps which show you how to calculate daily allowance of cholesterol and fats. Then you should use the worksheet following that to arrive at the daily calories, cholesterol, and percent of fats in your own diet. The following examples of daily food intake show the total calorie intake then figure the percent of total daily fats and saturated, monounsaturated, and polyunsaturated fat intake.

EXAMPLE 1

A person who eats an average 2,000 calories a day

Total Daily Calorie Intake: 2,000

Total Daily Cholesterol Allowance: 250–300 mg

Total Daily Fat Calorie Allowance = 30% of total calories or $.30 \times 2,000 = 600$ calories

Total Daily Fat Grams Allowance = $600/9 = 66.6$ grams of fat

Maximum Saturated Fat: less than 10% of the total calories

Actual Saturated Fat Calories (8%) = $.08 \times 2,000 = 160$

Actual Saturated Fat Grams = $160/9 = 17.7$

Maximum Monounsaturated Fat: 15% of total calories

Actual Monounsaturated Fat Calories (15%)
= $.15 \times 2,000 = 300$

Actual Monounsaturated Fat Grams = 300/9 = 33.3

Maximum Polyunsaturated Fat: less than 10% of the total calories

Actual Polyunsaturated Fat Calories (7%) = .07 × 2,000 = 140

Actual Polyunsaturated Fat Grams = 140/9 = 15.5

EXAMPLE 2

A person who eats an average of 1,600 calories a day

Total Daily Calorie Intake: 1,600

Total Daily Cholesterol Allowance: 250–300 mg

Total Daily Fat Calorie Allowance = 30% of total calories or .30 × 1,600 = 480 calories

Total Daily Fat Grams Allowance = 480/9 = 53.3 grams of fat

Maximum Saturated Fat: less than 10% of the total calories

Actual Saturated Fat Calories (6%) = .06 × 1,600 = 96

Actual Saturated Fat Grams = 96/9 = 10.6

Maximum Monounsaturated Fat: 15% of total calories

Actual Monounsaturated Fat Calories (15%) = .15 × 1,600 = 240

Actual Monounsaturated Fat Grams = 240/9 = 26.6

Maximum Polyunsaturated Fat: less than 10% of the total calories

Actual Polyunsaturated Fat Calories (7%) = .07 × 1,600 = 112

Actual Polyunsaturated Fat Grams = 112/9 = 12.4

EXAMPLE 3

A person who eats an average of 3,000 calories a day

Total Daily Calorie Intake: 3,000

Total Daily Cholesterol Allowance: 250–300 mg

Total Daily Fat Calorie Allowance = 30% of total calories or .30 × 3,000 = 900 calories

Total Daily Fat Grams Allowance = 900/9 = 100 grams of fat

Maximum Saturated Fat: less than 10% of the total calories

Actual Saturated Fat Calories (10%) = .10 × 3,000 = 300

Actual Saturated Fat Grams = 300/9 = 33.3

Maximum Monounsaturated Fat: 15% of total calories

Actual Monounsaturated Fat Calories (15%) = .15 × 3,000 = 450

Actual Monounsaturated Fat Grams = 450/9 = 50

Maximum Polyunsaturated Fat: less than 10% of the total calories

Actual Polyunsaturated Fat Calories (5%) = .05 × 3,000 = 150

Actual Polyunsaturated Fat Grams = 150/9 = 16.6

To use the worksheet to calculate your own daily calorie total, fat calorie total, saturated fat total, unsaturated fat total, and daily cholesterol intake, follow the steps listed below.

STEP 1

Keep a running list of everything you eat throughout the entire day. Write everything on this log so that you will get into the habit of recording. Use package labels or calorie-counter books to determine the calories, fat, saturated fat, and cholesterol. Add up the numbers for each meal and each snack.

STEP 2

To find the unsaturated fat in a food, use the label to find the total fat and subtract the saturated fat (listed on the label) from the total. This answer will give you the amount of unsaturated fat.

STEP 3

At the bottom of the sheet, add all meals and snacks together to arrive at the daily total.

STEP 4

Now that you know the total calorie count and total fat count, you will work to find what percentage of the calories came from fat. The daily total fat allowance in calories should not exceed 30%. Take your total calories for the day and multiply it by .30.

STEP 5

If the number you have recorded for the total fat is greater than the number you just got by multiplying the daily calories by .30, then you are eating more than the recommended maximum of 30% of total calories from fat. You will need to make adjustments in your diet to reduce the total fat calories to less than 30%.

STEP 6

Look at the saturated fat calories. Are they greater than 10% of your total calorie intake? To find out, multiply the total calorie number by .10. If the number you recorded for saturated fat exceeds the number you just got by multiplying .10 by the total calories, you are eating too much saturated fat. If the number is less than 10%, congratulations! You are already on your way to dietary control of your cholesterol.

STEP 7

Add all of the cholesterol intake recorded for the entire day to arrive at the total daily cholesterol intake. This number should be less than 300 mg to stay within the guidelines.

DAILY CHOLESTEROL AND FAT ALLOWANCE WORKSHEET
(Unsaturated fats include polyunsaturated and
monounsaturated)

Breakfast:

Food	Calories	Total Fat	Sat.	Unsat.	Chol.

Total: _____ _____ ____ _____ _____

Lunch:

Food	Calories	Total Fat	Sat.	Unsat.	Chol.

Total: _____ _____ ____ _____ _____

Dinner:

Food	Calories	Total Fat	Sat.	Unsat.	Chol.

Total: _____ _____ ____ _____ _____

Snacks:

Food	Calories	Total Fat	Sat.	Unsat.	Chol.
Total:	_____	_____	____	_____	_____

Meal	Calories	Total Fat	Sat.	Unsat.	Chol.
Breakfast	_____	_____	____	_____	_____
Lunch	_____	_____	____	_____	_____
Dinner	_____	_____	____	_____	_____
Snacks	_____	_____	____	_____	_____
Daily Total	_____	_____	____	_____	_____

6 Reading and Understanding Labels

This chapter will concentrate on providing guidelines to help in the process of selecting low-cholesterol and low-saturated-fat food choices. In the first five chapters you have learned what cholesterol is, where it comes from, and how the body utilizes it. You have also learned about the different types of cholesterol and how each type either accelerates or retards atherosclerosis and heart disease. The recommended daily allowances for dietary intake of fats and cholesterol as well as the normal and recommended blood levels have also been discussed. *Since dietary control is the key to the entire issue of conquering cholesterol,* it is extremely important that you be able to apply this information in a practical way. Now it is time to put all of your cholesterol knowledge to work for you. In this chapter, you will learn how to make wise low-fat selections based on food groups in combination with reading and interpreting labels.

In selecting any food, you want to consider its cholesterol, saturated and unsaturated fat content.

Saturated fats actually have *more* effect on the blood cholesterol level than does dietary cholesterol. The best dietary control of your cholesterol requires limiting foods high in cholesterol and saturated fats. Reducing your intake of saturated fat will be a start to controlling cholesterol, but additionally you will have to keep your total fat intake to less than 30% of your total daily calorie intake. This 30% must also be in the proper proportions to achieve good dietary control of your blood cholesterol profile. We will start with some broad guidelines for categories of food. Vegetable sources of food, with the exception of palm and coconut products, are always lower cholesterol choices than animal products. If you are choosing animal products, fish is the best choice. Turkey and chicken without the skin are the next best. (Remember to remove the skin from the turkey and chicken, because that is where the largest amount of cholesterol and saturated fat is contained.) When choosing beef, pork, lamb, or veal, remove as much fat as possible before cooking. If you cook with the fat on the meat, the fat will be absorbed into the meat. Trimming fat after cooking is not an efficient way to be in control of cholesterol.

Dairy products are also a source of cholesterol and saturated fat. There are now many no-fat dairy substitutes. The no-fat dairy substitutes include, but are not limited to, no-fat cheeses, sour cream, coffee creamers, cream cheese, cottage cheese, skim milk, .5% milk, and non-fat yogurt. Low-fat dairy foods include mozzarella cheese, buttermilk, and ice milk. These low-fat products would be good choices as well as substitutions for the dairy products you currently use. Dairy products moderately high in cholesterol and saturated fats include 1% or 2% milk, low-fat cottage cheese, and yogurt. Dairy products that are high in cholesterol and saturated fat include whole milk, creamed cottage cheese, and ice cream. These products should be avoided or limited. Egg yolks are the highest source of dietary cholesterol available. All of the cholesterol in an egg is contained in the yolk.

With these general guidelines in mind, we will now interpret some product labels. For most products with high cholesterol and/or high saturated fat content, there is usually a low-cholesterol, low-saturated fat, or no-fat substitute available. It will take time for you to find substitution products that appeal to your sense of taste, but it can be done. Remember, dietary control is the key to conquering cholesterol and that begins with awareness of what you eat.

LABELS

Reading food labels and understanding the information on them will help you conquer cholesterol and make wise food choices. Although there is a lot of information on a label, which can be confusing, this information can help you control your cholesterol.

In May of 1994, new labeling laws went into effect in the United States. These new label laws make reading the content of food much easier. While the new labels certainly help make the job easier, it is still ultimately your responsibility to not only read the label but to then interpret it. You must determine if that particular food or product fits into your personal low-fat diet plan. As already discussed, low cholesterol content and proper amounts of saturated and unsaturated fats are best for controlling your cholesterol level.

Food labels generally contain three types of information: (1) the ingredients, (2) nutritional facts, and (3) descriptive labeling terms. Some labels, for various reasons, still do not include all three types of information. When partial information is supplied, it will require you to more thoroughly investigate the label.

Products that only list ingredients use the minimum labeling. If that is the only information supplied by the manufacturer, it will be up to you to use that list to help understand the fat and cholesterol content of the food.

The ingredient portion of the label lists from highest content to lowest content. That is, the first ingredient is present in the largest amount, and the last ingredient is present in the least amount. That means that if a margarine product lists liquid corn oil, partially hydrogenated corn oil, and water as its ingredients, the product contains mostly liquid corn oil. Partially hydrogenated corn oil is the second most prevalent and water is the least prevalent ingredient.

It is best for unsaturated fats to be present in a larger quantity than saturated fats. Always keep in mind the 30% rule. That is, 30% or less of daily calories is the maximum allowable fat intake. Scrutinize labels and limit your saturated and hydrogenated fat intake. As unsaturated fats are better than saturated fats, so are partially hydrogenated fats better than hydrogenated fats.

By knowing the ingredients, you can make wise cholesterol and fat choices with the limited nutritional information provided on the label. Pay attention to the ingredient list, remembering that the contents are listed from the greatest volume to the least volume. This is true for all labels, even those supplying detailed nutritional information. Knowing that ingredients are always listed in this manner may provide you with a way to practice how accurate you can be at determining saturated, monounsaturated, andpolyunsaturated fats in any given food.

Using a label that gives all of the nutritional values, try covering the facts portion and using only the ingredient list. Then look at the actual label to determine how close you came to guessing correctly. This can be an invaluable tool to help you gain an appreciation of fat content. For instance, if you are in a restaurant and a description of the item is listed, see how close you can come to guessing the fat content or, more importantly, the types of fat. You will not be able to determine the exact amount of any given fat, but you will appreciate whether the fat is saturated and if there is a prevalence of a particular type of fat.

The nutritional facts are the second type of information provided by the food label, including the calorie content. This information is useful to help obtain and maintain ideal body weight. (Obtaining and maintaining ideal body weight is discussed in detail in Chapters 9 and 10.) With the nutritional facts provided on the food label, it is much less complicated to accurately interpret labels.

One of the biggest changes in the 1994 label laws was in the nutritional information section. The total fat is listed along with the amount of saturated fat. The cholesterol content is listed along with several other nutritionally important pieces of information. The remaining information is important from a balanced diet point of view, but not as a direct means for controlling fat or cholesterol. These additional nutritional factors include sodium, total carbohydrates, dietary fiber, sugar, protein, and vitamins and minerals.

Let's concentrate on the total fat, saturated fat, and cholesterol portions of the label since they will be the values you will want to consider when controlling your cholesterol. Two values are given for each category. To help you better understand these two values, let's examine each of them.

Total fat is given first as the total amount of fat (all fat) in a single serving of that food. Keeping in mind your total daily calorie intake, calculate the total grams of fat that you would maximally be allowed each day. The total fat will then be expressed as a percent of the daily value. This is an important number to interpret correctly. Remember that you want your maximum daily total of fat to be less than 30% of total calories. The percent of the daily value expressed on the label is usually based on a 2,000-calorie diet. If you eat something other than 2,000 calories daily, you must calculate what percent of your calorie intake that particular food represents. Do not use the percent of daily value without comparing it to your own particular calorie intake. The same method is used for displaying the saturated fat in a product. A total saturated fat per serving will appear, and also a percent of daily calories (again based on 2,000-calorie-a-day intake). These numbers are a good place to start your analysis, but remember to make the calculations, as discussed in Chapter 5, to reflect your personal eating habits.

The cholesterol is listed in milligrams (mg). Remember, your total daily intake of cholesterol should be 250–300 mg or less per day. All of the nutritional information is given for a specific serving size. That serving size is the first piece of information listed on the new labels. Pay attention to the serving size and adjust your interpretation of the label to your own serving size. If you use more than the listed serving portion, you must multiply the information; if you use less, you must divide the nutritional information to accurately reflect your intake. For example, if you use a mayonnaise that contains 20 mg of cholesterol per tablespoon, and you use two tablespoons, you are ingesting 40 mg of cholesterol ($2 \times 20 = 40$).

We have just discussed the nutritional facts portion of the label and explained how to interpret the information found there. But as you well know, that is not the only part of the label to contain information about the fat and cholesterol content. There are descriptive terms that are used for advertising purposes. These advertising terms were not subject to Food and Drug Administration (FDA) regulations prior to the labeling act of 1994. Now, advertisers can not label a product as "LOW FAT," unless it meets government-approved conditions. You will find a complete listing of the descriptive labeling terms approved by the FDA in Table 6.1. The descriptive terms used to define the fat and cholesterol content of foods must adhere precisely to the regulations imposed by the FDA. For example, the terms NO-FAT, FAT-FREE, or ZERO FAT all mean the same thing by definition. And that definition is that the product contains less than 0.5 grams of fat in each serving. You will have to refer to the nutritional facts portion of the label to determine the fat content of the serving size of that particular product. Descriptive terms have proven to be a source of very confusing advertising with questionable truths in years past. Now, with the approved descriptive labeling terms required by the FDA, the mystery is taken out of even the advertising portion of the label. This is good news for you, the conscientious and discriminating shopper. To take control of cholesterol and heart disease, you will need to examine all the information provided on the label. A little practice makes this seemingly difficult task much easier than you might presently suspect.

Let's start with how to interpret the information by examining a sample product label. After reviewing this label, we will compare different labels for similar foods. These foods will have different cholesterol and

Table 6.1 Descriptive Labeling Terms Approved by FDA: A Translation to Components Important in a Cholesterol-Lowering Diet

Nutrient	Free	Low	Reduced/ Less/Fewer	Other
All	Synonyms for "Free": "Free of," "No," "Zero," "Without," "Trivial Source of," "Negligible Source of," "Dietary Insignificant Source of"	Synonyms for "Low": "Contains a Small Amount of," "Low Source of," "Low in"	Synonyms for "Reduced/ Less/Fewer": "Reduced in," "Lower," "Low"	— —
Total calories	Less than 5 calories/ reference serving	Less than 40 calories/ reference serving	Reduced by at least 25%	
Total fat	Less than 0.5 g/ reference serving	3 g or less/reference serving Meal and main dish products: 3 g or less per 100 g product and 30% or less calories from fat	Reduced by at least 25%	" % Fat Free," " % Lean," must meet requirements for "low-fat"

Saturated fat	Less than 0.5 g/reference serving, levels of trans fatty acids must be 1% or less of total fat	1 g or less/reference serving and 15% or less of calories from saturated fatty acids Meal and main dish products: 1 g or less per 100 g, and less than 10% of calories from saturated fat	Reduced by at least 25%	
Cholesterol	Less than 2 mg/reference serving; saturated fat content must be 2 g or less	20 mg or less/reference serving; saturated fat content must be 2 g or less per serving Meal and main dish products: 20 mg or less per 100 g, with saturated fat content less than 2 g/100 g	Reduced by at least 25% Contains 2 g or less saturated fat per reference serving	
Sodium	Less than 5 mg/reference serving	140 mg or less/reference serving Meal and main dish products: 140 mg or less/100 g of food	Reduced by at least 25%	"Very Low Sodium," "Very Low in Sodium": 35 mg or less/reference serving

fat content or different polyunsaturated:saturated fat ratios. This exercise will help prepare you for making wise food choices to control cholesterol.

SAMPLE LABELS

Campbell's Tomato Soup

Serving Size:	½ Cup (120 ml) condensed soup
Calories:	100
Fat Calories:	20
Total Fat:	2 g 3% Daily Value
Saturated Fat:	0 g 0% Daily Value
Cholesterol:	0 mg 0% Daily Value

INGREDIENTS: Tomato puree (water, tomato paste), water, high fructose corn syrup, wheat flour, salt, vegetable oil (corn, cottonseed, or partially hydrogenated soybean oil), spice extract, vitamin C (ascorbic acid), and citric acid

As you begin your examination of this label, you will see that in the nutritional information provided, we elected not to include the breakdown of sodium, carbohydrates, protein, or vitamins and minerals. (This will be true for all label analysis in this book.) These nutritional ingredients were not included because they do not affect the blood cholesterol. However, they are important when considering the entire picture of good, balanced nutrition.

Let's examine the nutritional facts portion of the Campbell's soup label first. It is pretty straightforward that this would be considered a good low fat-choice. First of all, the total fat is 2 g. This contributes only 3% of the total fat in a 2,000-calorie diet. Remember, depending on the total number of daily calories you consume, this percentage may change. Further examination of the label reveals that there is no saturated fat and no cholesterol in this product. That is good news on two fronts. This all looks pretty clear, but is there anything that we missed? Yes! Look back to the serving size part of the label. It is listed as ½ cup or 120 ml of condensed soup. But do you eat this product as condensed soup? The answer is usually no. Because the nutritional information does not consider the diluent, you must. If you use water, which is one suggestion on the label, the nutritional information will remain unchanged. Water contains no fat, cholesterol, or calories. What if you use skim milk, which is another suggestion for preparation? How will this change the nutritional information? You would have to include skim milk in addition to the condensed soup, for accuracy. Looking at the skim milk label, we see that the serving size is 8 fluid ounces or 240 ml. There are 80 calories in each serving, and the calories from fat are 0; therefore the saturated fat is also 0. There is less than 5 mg of cholesterol per serving, which is 1% of the daily value for cholesterol on a 2,000-calorie diet.

Now that we have included the diluent in our analysis, is there anything else to consider? The answer again is yes. Look at the serving size for the skim milk. The information given is for 8 fluid ounces. If we look at the suggestions on the can, it says to add one can of water or skim milk to the condensed soup. A can is 10¾, not 8 ounces. You will have to adjust the calorie intake to reflect the additional skim milk used in the preparation of the soup. This does not add fat or saturated fat, but it will add more cholesterol. While the additional calories and cholesterol in this particular product are not terribly significant, it is easy to see that label reading is not always as simple as it appears.

Even in the face of the new labeling laws, you must be an astute consumer.

With so many products that come in a low- or no-fat choice, as well as the original version, we thought it would be helpful to compare a couple labels. We have used the same brand of original and "low-fat" versions for our comparisons.

Kraft Real Mayonnaise

Nutritional Facts

Serving Size:	1 tablespoon (14 g)
Calories:	100
Fat Calories:	100
Total Fat:	11 g 17% Daily Value
Saturated Fat:	2 g 10% Daily Value
Cholesterol:	10 mg 3% Daily Value

One of the first things that you observe when analyzing this label is that all of the calories come from fat. The total fat is 11 g, which is 17% of the total fat allowed each day on a 2,000-calorie diet. This is a large portion of your daily allowance in just a tablespoon of a product. The second piece of information that you notice is that there are 2 g of saturated fat, and this is 10% of your total daily allowance of saturated fat. Remember saturated fat is the type that promotes atherosclerosis and heart disease. Additionally there are 10 mg of cholesterol, or 3% of your daily allotment of cholesterol.

Let's look at the Kraft Free, Nonfat Mayonnaise Dressing for a comparasion.

Kraft Free, Nonfat Mayonnaise Dressing

Nutritional Facts

Serving Size:	1 tablespoon (16 g)
Calories:	10
Total Fat:	0 g 0% Daily Value
Saturated Fat:	0 g 0% Daily Value
Cholesterol:	0 mg 0% Daily Value

This product is a clear winner when looking at the nutritional information provided. There are only 10 calories as opposed to 100. None of the calories come from fat, whereas in the previous product all of the calories came from fat. Additionally, there is no fat or cholesterol in this product. From the perspective of trying to control your intake of fat, especially saturated fat and cholesterol, the Kraft Free, Nonfat Mayonnaise Dressing is the obvious choice.

You may ask yourself, how can they do that? How can a product that contained 100 calories, all from fat, with 11 g of total fat and 2 g of saturated fat make it disappear? The truth of the matter is in the ingredient portion of the label. By examining the ingredients, we can really see how a company can make a similar product with a lot less fat or sometimes no fat. To fully understand this, we will look at the ingredient list on both of these labels.

Kraft Real Mayonnaise

INGREDIENTS: Soybean oil, eggs, vinegar, water, egg yolks, salt, sugar, pure lemon juice concentrate, dried garlic, dried onion, calcium disodium EDTA as a preservative, paprika, natural flavor.

Kraft Free, Nonfat Mayonnaise Dressing

INGREDIENTS: Water, sugar, food starch-modified, natural flavor, contains less than 2% of cellulose gel, vinegar, salt, dried corn syrup, lactic acid, artificial color, potassium sorbate, and calcium disodium EDTA as preservatives, cream*, lemon juice concentrate, phosphoric acid, skim milk, paprika, egg yolks*, vitamin E, xanthan gum, mustard flour, dried garlic, dried onion, beta carotene, yellow 6, blue 1.

The first rule to remember when analyzing the ingredient list is that ingredients are listed from the most prevalent to the least prevalent by volume. Right away we can see that the most prevalent ingredient in the real mayonnaise is soybean oil. You already know that soybean oil is a polyunsaturated fat. The first ingredient listed on the nonfat mayonnaise dressing is water. It is obvious from reading the ingredient list why one product contains fat and the other is a nonfat alternative. As you continue to analyze the ingredients in the real mayonnaise, you will find eggs, a source of cholesterol, as the second ingredient. The fifth ingredient is egg yolks. As we discussed before, all of the cholesterol in an egg is found in the yolk. So the ingredient list on this product informs you that there is cholesterol from the eggs and additional cholesterol from the yolks. By comparison, the second label has water listed as its first ingredient, and this certainly does not contain fat or cholesterol. In fact you have to go all the way to the thirteenth ingredient to find any fat source at all. And the cream is identified as being a trivial source of fat in this product, as described in the standards set down by the FDA. The only source of choles-

---

* trivial source of fat and cholesterol.

terol in this product is found as ingredient eighteen, egg yolks. And again it is noted that the amount of egg yolks used in this particular product is a trivial amount and therefore not considered enough to affect the blood cholesterol. By examining the nutritional facts portion of the food label, you were able to clearly see which product offered a low-fat alternative. By further examination of the label to include the ingredient list, you were able to see how the company produced a no-fat substitute. Do not limit your label reading to the nutritional facts portion; also examine the ingredient list, the preparation suggestions, and the serving size to get the whole story.

Next we will examine two more products, one a reduced fat and one the original.

LABEL #1

Jif Creamy Peanut Butter

Serving Size:	2 tablespoons	
Calories:	190	
Total Fat:	16 g	25% Daily Value
Saturated Fat:	3 g	16% Daily Value
Cholesterol:	0 mg	

INGREDIENTS: Roasted peanuts and sugar. Contains 2% or less of: molasses, partially hydrogenated vegetable oil (soybean), fully hydrogenated vegetable oils (rapeseed and soybean), mono- and diglycerides, and salt.

LABEL #2

Jif Reduced Fat Creamy Peanut Spread

Serving Size: 2 tablespoons

Calories:	190	
Total Fat:	12 g	18% Daily Value
Saturated Fat:	2 g	10% Daily Value
Cholesterol:	0 mg	

INGREDIENTS: Peanuts, corn syrup solids, sugar, soy protein. Contains 2% or less of: fully hydrogenated vegetable oils (rapeseed and soybean), salt, mono- and diglycerides, molasses, niacinamide, folic acid, pyridoxine hydrochloride, magnesium oxide, zinc oxide, ferric orthophosphate, and copper sulfate

You can see by comparing these two products that the fat content was reduced from 16 g total fat to 12 g total fat. Even this seemingly small reduction in fat will go a long way in helping you control your cholesterol by controlling your dietary fat.

Interpreting the Label

It is best to get into the habit of reading food labels in the grocery store before you buy. If you read labels after the product is purchased, chances are you will eat the food even though you determine that it is high in cholesterol and/or saturated fat.

To repeat, there are three types of information on food labels: the nutritional facts, ingredient list, and descriptive labeling terms. Compare various food products to make the best low-cholesterol, low-saturated-fat choice. There are many products that you think are similar until you actually examine the label. Under the nutritional facts portion of the label, the serving size will be listed. All the remaining information given is dependent on the serving size, so pay attention and adjust according to your portions.

Practice, Practice, Practice

Reading labels may seem a bit frustrating and time consuming if you do not currently look at food labels critically. But, if you keep reading and practicing, it will soon become second nature to you. Since anything becomes easier with some practice, the next few pages are samples of actual food labels for you to interpret and compare. At the end of the examples, there are questions to see if you made the best choice available. There are also comments about how to arrive at the best choice. Don't worry, time and practice will make it easy for you to be the wise shopper your heart deserves. If you take the time now to examine what you eat, you will have the time later to enjoy good health.

The following are sample product labels. These are included in this chapter to give you some practice in interpretation. Interpret the labels by asking yourself: Does this product contain fat? Is that fat saturated or unsaturated? Is there cholesterol in this product?

Hearty Italian Tomato Sauce

Serving Size:	4 oz. (½ cup or 129 g)
Calories:	80
Total Fat:	3 g 5% Daily Value
Saturated Fat:	0.5 g 2% Daily Value
Cholesterol:	0 mg

INGREDIENTS: Tomatoes, soybean oil, salt, corn syrup, dried onions, Romano cheese made from cows' milk, olive oil, spices, garlic powder

When you examine the label for the Hearty Italian Tomato Sauce, you see that the cholesterol content, total fat, and saturated fat contents have all been provided for you. The last question—Does this product contain cholesterol?—is clearly answered for you. The answer is no. You can now address the question—Is there fat in this product, and if so, is it in the 2:1 ratio of polyunsaturated to saturated fat (P:S)? This is not specifically stated on the label so you will have to use the ingredient list to analyze the 3 grams of fat. Tomatoes are fruit so they do not contain saturated fats. Soybean oil is a polyunsaturated fat. It is better to have a fat in the liquid form (as it is in this product) than partially or completely hydrogenated. Salt, corn syrup, and dried onions are not considerations in regard to cholesterol and fat content. Romano cheese made from cows' milk will contain some butterfat. Olive oil is one of the monounsaturated fats and, therefore, is not a factor in determining P:S ratio. The two remaining ingredients (spices and garlic powder) do not contain fats. In examining this label you find that most of the 3 g will be either polyunsaturated (soybean oil) or monounsaturated (olive oil) with a small portion of the Romano cheese containing butterfat from the milk. This product would be a wise low-cholesterol, low-saturated-fat food choice.

Kellogg's Corn Flakes

Serving Size:	1 oz. (about 1 cup with ½ cup skim milk)
Calories:	110 cereal 150 with Skim Milk
Total Fat:	0 g 0% Daily Value
Saturated Fat:	0 g 0% Daily Value
Cholesterol:	0 mg

INGREDIENTS: Corn, sugar, salt, malt flavoring, corn syrup

The sample label for Kellogg's Corn Flakes shows that there is no fat and no cholesterol contained in this product. The dry cereal is a good food choice. If you choose to use whole milk instead of skim milk on your cereal, it will necessitate a reevaluation. Whole milk supplies an additional 30 calories, 4 g fat, and 15 mg of cholesterol.

Healthy Choice Low Fat Franks

Serving Size:	1 Frank (45 g)
Calories:	50
Fat Calories:	15
Total Fat:	1.5 g 2% Daily Value
Saturated Fat:	0.5 g 3% Daily Value
Cholesterol:	15 mg 5% Daily Value

INGREDIENTS: Turkey, turkey broth, pork, water, hydrolyzed milk protein, flavorings, dextrose, salt, starch (potato, modified corn), corn syrup, hydrolyzed oat flour, beef sodium lactate, vitamin C, sodium nitrate, extract of paprika

This label from low-fat franks is a good example of a how the nutritional facts, the ingredient list, and the descriptive label terms all work together. Turning first to the nutritional facts, you see that there are a small number of calories from fat and only 0.5 g of saturated fat. These values would certainly fit in a low-fat, low-cholesterol food plan. The ingredient list gives you the information that most of the calories and fat come from turkey, which is a lower-fat food choice. There is some pork but not as much as turkey. In examining the remaining ingredients, you find that there are no other fat sources in this product. Finally, using

Table 6.2   High-Cholesterol Foods

Foods High in Cholesterol

Liver	Sweetbreads
Heart	Gizzard
Kidneys	Brains
Chitterlings	Egg Yolk

Foods Moderately High in Cholesterol

Shrimp	Lobster
Sardines	Skin of Chicken and Turkey

Table 6.1, you see that the term low-fat franks fit within the guidelines. It is good to know that the label can be used in many ways to determine if you are making a good low-fat choice.

These examples have given you an opportunity to practice interpreting labels. Get into the habit of reviewing product labels before you buy so that you will have low-cholesterol, low-fat foods in your home. Look at all parts of the label. As you have seen, labels differ in the amount and type of information they provide. Examine the ingredient list and continue to look for all sources of fat and cholesterol in products. You should try to identify fats as polyunsaturated, saturated, and monounsaturated. Label interpretation will get easier with practice. It is well worth the time it takes to read labels so you bring good food home. By doing this, you will increase your chances of maintaining a healthy heart.

There are many low-cholesterol, low-saturated-fat food choices to substitute for those foods that promote heart disease. Tables 6.2, 6.3, and 6.4 are samples of foods that may help you make good low-fat, low-cholesterol choices.

Table 6.3 Substitutions

Column I	Column II
Whole Milk:	.5% Milk:
3.5% butterfat	0.5% butterfat
1 cup	1 cup
150 calories	90 calories
8 g total fat	1 g total fat
34 mg cholesterol	5 mg cholesterol
Butter:	Margarine:
1 tablespoon	1 tablespoon
12 g total fat	variable from 0 g to 11 g fat
35 mg cholesterol	0 mg cholesterol
Whole Egg:	Egg Substitute:
1 egg	2 oz. = 1 egg
80 calories	60 calories
6 g total fat	2 g total fat
213 mg cholesterol	0 mg cholesterol
Flavored Yogurt:	Non-Fat Plain Yogurt:
1 cup (8 oz.)	1 cup (8 oz.)
230 calories	150 calories
7 g total fat	0 g total fat
17 mg cholesterol	6 mg cholesterol
Creamed Cottage Cheese:	Low-Fat Cottage Cheese:
1 cup (8 oz.)	1 cup (8 oz.)
260 calories	170 calories
10 g total fat	1 g total fat
48 mg cholesterol	13 mg cholesterol
Ice cream:	No-Fat Frozen Dessert:
1 cup (8 oz.)	1 cup (8 oz.)
255 calories	100 calories
9 g total fat	0 g total fat
35 mg cholesterol	10 mg cholesterol

Table 6.4   Cholesterol Content of Meat and Meat Products

Food	Serving Size/Cholesterol
Fish (lean)	3 oz./63 mg
Chicken (skinless)	3 oz./74 mg
Turkey (skinless)	3 oz./74 mg
Cold Cuts	3 oz./82 mg
Beef Prime Rib	3 oz./85 mg
Hamburger (25% fat)	3 oz./85 mg
Veal Cutlet	3 oz./86 mg

7   Checking Lipid Levels

Determining your cholesterol level requires a blood test. A screening cholesterol test may be performed either fasting or non-fasting. The data show that total cholesterol levels are equally reliable in the fasting and non-fasting state. If a triglyceride level and the HDL cholesterol are being measured, then the blood specimen should be drawn after you have been fasting for a minimum of twelve hours. Most cholesterol levels are checked by having blood drawn from a vein (usually in the arm). The blood that is drawn can be checked for triglycerides and total cholesterol, as well as HDL, the good cholesterol component. The LDL cholesterol is usually not directly measured in the blood, but is calculated. The LDL cholesterol can be found by knowing the total cholesterol, triglycerides, and HDL cholesterol. This is sometimes referred to as an indirect measurement, because it is derived indirectly from the other known information. The formula for calculating the LDL cholesterol is:

LDL = Total Cholesterol − (Triglycerides/5) − HDL

For example, if your total cholesterol = 220, HDL = 45, and triglycerides = 125, your LDL cholesterol = 220 − (125/5) − 45 = 220 − 25 − 45 = 150.

Cholesterol is measured in milligrams (mg) in $\frac{1}{10}$ liter of blood (dL). For example, if your cholesterol level was reported to be 180 mg/dL, that would mean that every $\frac{1}{10}$ liter of your blood contains 180 mg of cholesterol. Mg/dL is the standard unit of cholesterol measurement in the U.S., but levels are generally spoken about (imprecisely) without the units or sometimes just as mgs. The recommendation from the National Institutes of Health (NIH) and the American Heart Association (AHA) is to reduce blood cholesterol to 200 mg/dL or less for all adults. The average blood cholesterol for Americans between the ages of 35 and 60 years was 211 mg/dL in 1984. The average blood cholesterol level in 1994 is thought to be approximately 205. That is a decrease from the average of 250 mg/dL in 1978. While these numbers show us that the trend in the United States is toward lower cholesterol levels, it is important to realize that the average cholesterol level of men who had a heart attack was 225 mg/dL. This is one of the reasons that the recommendation for the total cholesterol level is 200 mg/dL or less for all Americans over the age of two. There is a distinct difference between the "normal" level and the "recommended" level of blood cholesterol. The meaning of "normal" cholesterol level is based on the cholesterol level of a large number of Americans. A "mean value" and "standard deviation" are calculated from these values and the "normal levels" are thus determined. Unfortunately, because the American diet is high in cholesterol and saturated fats, the "normal levels" were determined to be quite high. The "recommended levels" are based on scientific studies that have shown at what level the risk of cardiovascular disease increases. Thus, the recommended levels are much lower than the previously accepted normal levels. For this reason the American Heart Association and the NIH have reevaluated the normal total cholesterol level for American adults. The current recommended normal of 200 mg/dL is to try to minimize the risk for heart disease. The first attempts at lowering cholesterol level to achieve the recommended value should always be dietary modifications. This is done by reducing the total cholesterol and saturated fat intake. The total intake of fats should be limited to 30%, with less than 10% from saturated fats, up to 10% from polyunsaturated, and 10–15% monounsaturated fats. The maximum daily cholesterol intake should be 250–300 mgs. If this diet is not successful in reaching the desired cholesterol level, a stricter diet containing less cholesterol and fat should be instituted. In addition, other dietary changes, such as decreasing calorie intake to obtain ideal body weight, should be employed. This and other ideas will be discussed in later chapters.

Everyone is encouraged to have his/her blood cholesterol level checked. You should be as aware of your cholesterol level as you are of your blood pressure. If the total cholesterol level is within the recommended limits (less than 200 mg/dL) and there are no other risk factors for heart disease present, the cholesterol can be checked every five years. If the total cholesterol is borderline-high at 200–239 mg/dL, there is a moderately increased risk of developing heart disease. At this cholesterol range, dietary modification should be made and the cholesterol level rechecked within one year. However, if there is coronary artery disease or two risk factors present, a lipid profile should be obtained. These risk factors include hypertension, smoking, family history of heart disease, being male, obesity, diabetes, history of peripheral vascular disease, or a low HDL cholesterol. Treatment and repeat cholesterol determinations would be based on the LDL cholesterol levels. (See Chapter 13 for more specific information.) If the cholesterol level is 240 mg/dL or above, the individual is considered to be in the high-risk category for developing coronary heart disease. A lipid profile should be obtained to help your personal physician prescribe dietary modifications and any necessary medication therapy. This will be at the discretion of your physician and will depend on the individual cholesterol level and overall risk factors.

If a person is in the high-risk category, the cholesterol level test should be repeated to confirm the abnormal results. The cholesterol level test should then be repeated as necessary to monitor dietary and/or medication effects. This can be done as frequently as once a month or, typically, every two to four months, until the desired levels are obtained. Cholesterol monitoring can then be done on a yearly basis or more frequently if your physician feels it is appropriate.

Because of the increased demands to have cholesterol level tests performed quickly, easily, and above all accurately, new techniques are being developed. Several machines are currently available that can determine a cholesterol level within minutes from blood obtained by a simple finger stick. This technique allows for mass screening of cholesterol in doctors' offices, work settings, clinics, health fairs, and now at home. Anyone with an elevated total cholesterol or abnormally high triglycerides should have a fasting specimen obtained for HDL cholesterol as well as for triglycerides.

BLOOD CHOLESTEROL LEVELS

Less than 200 mg/dL	Desirable
200–239 mg/dL	Borderline-high
Greater than or equal to 240 mg/dL	High

TRIGLYCERIDES

Triglycerides are another type of lipid in the blood. The role of triglycerides in the development and progression of atherosclerosis is currently not well defined. Medically little is known about triglycerides. What is known, however, is that elevation of the triglyceride level is frequently associated with cholesterol elevation. Triglycerides are not generally an independent factor in cardiovascular disease, but rather a predictor that other risk factors may be present. For instance, elevation of triglycerides is seen in association with obesity, diabetes, thyroid disease, and alcohol consumption, all of which increase the risk of cardiovascular disease. There is also some evidence that triglyceride levels increase with cigarette smoking and a sedentary lifestyle. Once again, both of these are risk factors for cardiovascular disease.

Triglyceride elevation, therefore, may signal other associated risk factors or be part of a larger problem of elevated total cholesterol. An elevated triglyceride level is an independent risk factor in women. Due to the fact that elevated triglyceride levels are associated with additional risks for coronary artery disease in men, and as an independent risk in women, the blood triglyceride level should be checked and monitored. The NIH consensus panel report recommended that triglycerides between 250 and 500 mg/dL should be used as a marker to carefully evaluate for other risk factors. The consensus panel further recommended that anyone with a triglyceride level above 500 mg/dL should be treated with diet and drug therapy. (See Chapter 13 for drug therapy.) The definitive answers to the role of triglycerides in the development and progression of atherosclerosis is not clear. But since there is an association between triglyceride elevation and cardiovascular disease, it is best to control the triglyceride blood level as well as the cholesterol level (see Chapter 3 for more information).

Types of Hyperlipidemia

As you remember from Chapter 2, the term lipid refers to any of the fats in the blood. The term hyperlipidemia simply means that one of the fats in the blood, either cholesterol or triglycerides, is elevated. The term hypercholesterolemia specifically means that the blood cholesterol level is elevated above the recommended levels. (The prefix "hyper" means increased or above normal.) As you have learned in the first part of this chapter, blood tests can directly measure the total cholesterol level, as well as HDL and triglycerides. From this information, the LDL cholesterol level can be calculated. When each category or specific lipid is analyzed, the exact cause for the high lipid level (hyperlipidemia) can be appreciated. Depending upon which component of the lipid profile is elevated, a specific name or type is given to that particular pattern of elevation. The simplified table that follows defines the types of hyperlipidemias and their arbitrary definitions (see Table 7.1). Type II is the most prevalent form of hypercholesterolemia found in the

Table 7.1 Classifications of Hyperlipidemia

	Cholesterol	Triglycerides	LDL	HDL
Type I	↑	↑↑↑	↓↓	↓↓
Type IIa	↑↑	—	↑↑	—
Type IIb	↑↑	↑	↑↑	↓
Type III	↑↑	↑↑	—	↓
Type IV	↑	↑↑	—	↓
Type V	↑↑	↑↑↑	↓	↓↓

↑   Small increase
↑↑ Moderate increase
↑↑↑ Large increase
—   Normal
↓   Small decrease
↓↓ Moderate decrease
↓↓↓ Large decrease

United States. Type II is divided into two categories: Type IIa and Type IIb.

Type IIa means that the total blood cholesterol is elevated and the triglycerides are normal. An elevation in the LDL cholesterol component is what causes an elevation in the total cholesterol. In other words, the person said to have Type IIa hypercholesterolemia has so much of the LDL, or bad cholesterol, that the total cholesterol is elevated. Type IIb hypercholesterolemia means that there is an elevation in the triglycerides as well as LDL cholesterol. The total cholesterol elevation is due to increased levels of LDL cholesterol and increased triglyceride levels. If we rearrange the formula previously used to calculate LDL, we see that:

Total Cholesterol = LDL + HDL + (triglycerides/5)

Therefore, an elevated triglyceride level will increase the measured total cholesterol blood level without necessarily increasing LDL level. Type IIa and IIb are the two most prevalent kinds of hypercholesterolemia. Both will respond to dietary management. Reducing the amount of saturated fats and cholesterol is the first step in the management of hypercholesterolemia. *Drugs are never a substitute for dietary control.* There are studies that show a diet high in saturated fats may actually override the effects of drugs used to lower cholesterol levels. In keeping with this same line of thinking, the amount of drug therapy necessary to control elevated cholesterol may be reduced with the addition of a low-fat, low-cholesterol diet.

The additional categories of hyperlipidemia are Type I, Type III, Type IV, and Type V. Because these types are much less common in the general population than Type II, they will not be discussed. The classifications were originally used for laboratory convenience only and have no relationship to the cause of the problem. Regardless of the specific type of hyperlipidemia you may have, it is important to remember that dietary control of saturated fats and cholesterol is the cornerstone to therapy. Without dietary modifications, it is impossible to effectively control any type of hyperlipidemia.

FACTORS THAT AFFECT BLOOD CHOLESTEROL LEVELS

In addition to the food you eat, several other factors will affect your blood cholesterol level. These include your weight, amount of exercise, whether and how much you smoke, your stress level, the amount of fiber and sugar in your diet, certain diseases, and some side effects of certain medications, especially medicines used to control high blood pressure. Also, an inherited genetic defect which affects the liver's ability to process cholesterol is found in about 1 in 500 people with elevated blood cholesterol levels. Obviously, other than an inherited genetic defect, most of these factors that affect cholesterol can be modified in a favorable manner.

The next chapter (Chapter 8) deals briefly with those diseases that have the most effect on the cholesterol level, as well as the medications that most commonly affect cholesterol as an undesirable side effect. In addition, fiber in the diet is discussed. These factors are less common and usually have less overall effect on the cholesterol blood level than does weight control, exercise, and smoking. Because of their importance, weight control, exercise, and smoking are discussed in more detail in Chapters 9 and 10.

8 Other Factors That Affect Lipids

There is a group of recognized factors, other than diet and genetic makeup, that can affect your blood cholesterol levels. Some of these factors are harmful and may raise the LDL cholesterol, whereas others, such as fiber intake, may actually help reduce cholesterol levels. First we will discuss the factors that can raise the blood cholesterol level. Cholesterol levels can increase as a result of some ailments such as hypothyroidism, diabetes, and some types of liver and kidney disease. This elevation of cholesterol is considered "secondary" because it happens as a result of a "primary" disease or problem. The treatment of choice of these secondary problems is to treat the underlying primary disease. It is important to re-emphasize at this point that, even if the cause of your elevated cholesterol is secondary to another problem, a low-cholesterol, low-saturated-fat diet is usually still recommended. This goes back to the fact that the normal American diet is too high in cholesterol and saturated fat. In addition to the above diseases, secondary elevation of blood cholesterol level can occur when taking certain medications. The following are some medications that have been extensively studied and proven to elevate cholesterol levels. Anabolic steroids and progesterones, particularly those which do not contain estrogens, are two medications that have been shown to elevate LDL cholesterol levels and drastically reduce HDL cholesterol. If these medications are necessary for the treatment of a disease or medical condition, they should be regulated by a physician. The cholesterol levels will then be checked during the course of drug therapy. These medications become particularly dangerous when individuals take them without the recommendation and follow-up of a physician. Anabolic steroids that are taken by athletes and bodybuilders without physician supervision may have very serious consequences by possibly accelerating atherosclerosis, which can lead to heart attack or stroke. Anabolic steroids have been shown to reduce the HDL cholesterol by as much as 10 to 70%. Studies of the effects of progesterones show a decrease in HDL cholesterol of 5 to 15%.

Some medications that are used in the treatment of hypertension raise total cholesterol. They do this by raising the LDL cholesterol and triglycerides while decreasing the beneficial HDL cholesterol. Medications that are used in the treatment of hypertension must be carefully regulated by a physician. Persons taking these medications should not discontinue or reduce the dosage without the consent of a physician. The possibility of suffering a stroke or heart attack from uncontrolled hypertension is high. The beneficial effects of controlling hypertension with certain medications must be weighed against their detrimental side effect of elevating the cholesterol level. Specifically, several diuretics (water pills) used to treat hypertension can elevate cholesterol levels. They raise LDL cholesterol levels and triglycerides as well as lower HDL cholesterol levels. Beta blockers are another type of anti-hypertensive medication that affects the cholesterol. Beta blockers elevate triglycerides and lower HDL cholesterol levels. The beta blockers usually have more effect on the blood cholesterol levels than the diuretics. Remember, medications are not to be discontinued or altered without the recommendation of your physician.

Diabetes is a risk factor, independent of elevated cholesterol, for coronary heart disease. In diabetes there is a change in the way fats are used by the body, along with a tendency to have an increased serum triglyceride level. Alterations are also seen in the blood vessels of diabetics. Because of the high risk associated with diabetes, specific recommendations have been written for this group of people. The recommendations from the NIH Cholesterol Adult Treatment Panel Report states that men with diabetes should lower their LDL cholesterol to less than 130 mg/dL and women to less than 160 mg/dL. If the woman has other risk factors for heart disease, the LDL should be reduced to 130 mg/dL. Some of these additional risk factors are hypertension, smoking, and family history of heart disease. For men and women with known atherosclerotic disease (coronary artery disease, carotid artery disease, or peripheral vascular disease), the recommended LDL level is less than 100 mg/dL. The same dietary plan is recommended for diabetics as for the general population (see Chapter 5).

If you have hypothyroidism, obstructive liver disease, or kidney disease, you should talk with your physician about your cholesterol levels. Be aware that all of these conditions may affect your cholesterol. The specifics of your particular condition will dictate a course of treatment for you. Remember, the first step in lowering your cholesterol level is to follow the diet changes discussed in this book.

What is the role of fiber in reducing cholesterol levels? There are two types of fiber: insoluble and soluble. The insoluble fiber has no affect on cholesterol. This type of fiber is the indigestible carbohydrate found in an average diet. An example of an insoluble fiber is cellulose, which is found in wheat bran and celery. Insoluble fiber adds bulk to the stool but does nothing to lower cholesterol levels. The second type of fiber is soluble and has been shown to lower cholesterol levels. This fiber is soluble (dissolves) in the intestine but is not absorbed. Some examples of soluble fiber are pectins, certain gums, and psyllium. Pectins are found in many fruits, and one of the beneficial gums is found in oats and beans. Psyllium is the ingredient in Metamucil that has been shown to reduce cholesterol. Studies have shown that taking 15 to 25 grams of soluble fiber each day lowers total cholesterol by 5% to 15%. Some people have gastrointestinal irritability with this amount of fiber, but it appears that, with long-term use, the side effects will frequently diminish.

9   Exercise

A major goal of cholesterol control is to achieve and maintain ideal body weight according to the guidelines set down by the National Cholesterol Education Program of the National Institutes of Health. It has become apparent that the number of overweight people in this country is growing at an alarming rate based on several recent national studies. People who are overweight have many potential health problems, including an increased risk of cardiovascular disease. Overweight is now considered a national health crisis. In the period between 1988 and 1991, 33.4% of the U.S. population over the age of 20 were estimated to be overweight. This is an increase of 8% from the previous survey. There are several consequences of an overweight society, and this becomes very apparent when you consider the health costs. *The economics of health care costs associated with overweight are in excess of $39 billion.*

OVERWEIGHT

This increase in health costs relating to overweight, combined with the prevalence of cardiovascular disease in the United States, are two reasons that the federal health authorities have targeted reducing overweight as one of its primary objectives. To help meet this objective, the Healthy People 2000 Program was initiated by the U.S. Department of Health and Human Services (USDHHS). USDHHS is working toward the goal of increased fitness in the general population of the country by the year 2000. Some of the goals of Healthy People 2000 are:

- Reduce coronary heart disease deaths and the prevalence of overweight.
- Increase moderate daily physical activity and cardiorespiratory fitness.
- Reduce the number of people leading sedentary lifestyles.
- Increase muscular strength, endurance, and flexibility.
- Improve diet and physical activity habits among the overweight.
- Increase daily participation in physical education in schools.
- Increase worksite physical activity and fitness programming.
- Increase community physical activity and fitness facilities.
- Increase physical activity counseling by primary care givers.

A two-part approach must be undertaken to successfully reduce overweight. The first necessary step is the sensible use of a low-fat diet and decreased calorie intake. But this must be combined with a routine exercise program that will lead to ideal body weight and, more particularly, ideal body composition. We have discussed the low-fat diet in Chapter 5 with regard to the Step I diet, and ideal body weight will be discussed under the section titled "Obtaining and Maintaining Ideal Body Weight" in Chapter 10. We will now take a look at exercise, the second part of the plan to reduce weight.

Exercise is an essential part of the total plan to improve your cholesterol status and help reduce your risk of heart disease. Numerous studies have shown that regular physical exercise increases the amount of HDL (good) cholesterol and lowers the LDL (bad) cholesterol and triglycerides. Not only does regular exercise improve the cholesterol profile, but a sedentary lifestyle is one of the risk factors for coronary heart disease. In fact, a sedentary lifestyle was one of the strongest predictors of coronary heart disease in the 1988 Behavior Risk Factor Surveillance System data from the Center for Disease Control (CDC). The Surveillance System assessed the prevalence of a sedentary lifestyle at 58%. That compares to the prevalence of smoking at 25%, obesity at 22%, hypertension at 17%, and diabetes at 5%, using the CDC Behavior Risk Factor Surveillance System.

To help ensure your success with undertaking an exercise regimen, you should consider several things. One major consideration for a successful exercise program is the realization that exercise must be something that you can and should do forever. Exercise is not a six-week or twelve-month program, but a lifelong commitment. This is no different than the routine obligation to brushing your teeth or shampooing your hair. Because exercise is for life, it is important to choose an activity that you enjoy. In this way, you will find the exercise easier to do and will be more likely to continue it indefinitely. If you dislike walking, don't start a walking program.

Many activities are beneficial to the cardiovascular system, and these will help increase your HDL cholesterol. Choose activities that are best suited for you and your lifestyle. It may be best to choose two or three different activities. In that way, you may minimize the boredom factor and increase the chance that you will continue the activities long term. You should consult your physician before starting any exercise program if you have not been physically active. To gain cardiovascular benefits, exercise should be done at least three times a week for a minimum of 20 minutes each session. The excuse that you don't have time for a regular exercise program is a poor one. Isn't your life and health worth 45–60 minutes a week? Start slowly! It will take time to build your endurance. You may not be able to exercise for 15–20 minutes continuously the first time you try, but keep at it. Anything is better than being a couch potato.

AEROBIC EXERCISE

Exercises that are particularly good for your cardiovascular health and cholesterol levels are those that are said to be aerobic in nature. You may be asking yourself what is meant by aerobic exercise and what kinds of exercises are aerobic. Let us start with defining aerobic exercise. Aerobic means that the presence of oxygen is required. Oxygen is used to produce a chemical in the body known as ATP. Active muscles in the body convert carbohydrates and fatty acids to ATP to achieve muscle contraction. Because the large muscles of the body are working hard to contract during aerobic exercise, a lot of carbohydrates and fatty acids are used. Blood that is rich in oxygen must be delivered to the muscles during exercise. It is the oxygen from the blood that provides the muscles with the oxygen needed to produce ATP.

It is easy to see that aerobic exercise depends on the interaction of the cardiovascular (heart and blood vessels) and respiratory systems (lungs) of the body. The work that is done by the cardiovascular and respiratory systems during exercise helps keep the heart and lungs healthy. The conversion of carbohydrates and fatty acids to ATP helps reduce and/or maintain a healthy weight. This is why aerobic exercise will help your cardiovascular health and aid in maintaining or achieving an ideal weight.

Now that you know what an aerobic activity is, you are probably trying to identify some examples. Walking, swimming, jogging, bicycling, dancing, in-line skating, rope jumping, and cross-country skiing are all great examples of aerobic exercise. To be more successful in starting and staying with an aerobic activity program, you will want to incorporate a warm-up and cool-down segment. Warm-ups and cool-downs benefit the cardiovascular, respiratory, and muscular systems. Many people warm up before an activity, just because it is usually more comfortable to do so; but often cooling down is neglected. Cooling down and stretching after aerobic activity can help minimize soreness. Lactic acid is a by-product produced by muscles when they work. If the lactic acid is not removed from the muscle following activity, it can form tiny crystals in the muscle. These crystals irritate the muscle and cause soreness. You can decrease or prevent this from happening by stretching and cooling down after exercise. The stretch will increase blood flow to the muscle fibers and gently wash out the lactic acid that has formed. Decreasing the lactic acid left in the muscle means fewer crystals will be formed, and that translates to less soreness in the days following an activity. In addition to the muscular benefits, warming up and cooling down helps ease the heart and lungs into and out of a more active working role.

Remember that whatever activity you choose, it should be one that you can do for 15–20 minutes continuously. Choose activities that are enjoyable to you and fit your lifestyle. For example, if you have knee problems, the non-weight-bearing activity of swimming or water aerobics may be best for you. However, if you do not have access to a pool, it would be foolish to consider water aerobics as your primary activity. Consistency is an important part of whatever physical activity program you choose, so start today and stay with it for life!

10 Take Control of Your Cholesterol

Chest pain, heart attack, and stroke can have a devastating effect on your life. Do you want these problems to be part of your future? If not, it is up to you to do *all* that you can to prevent them. In addition to lowering your LDL cholesterol and triglycerides and raising your HDL cholesterol, you may have to make other changes. But isn't life worth it? We have spent a large portion of this book explaining why controlling cholesterol is important. The best way to lower cholesterol is to reduce total fat intake and limit saturated fat and cholesterol. These in fact are the guidelines set by the American Heart Association. In addition, obtaining and maintaining ideal body weight and composition, adhering to a regular exercise program, stopping smoking, and taking lipid-lowering drugs as prescribed by your physician also help control your cholesterol. You have learned about cholesterol and fat intake. The previous chapter exclusively examined exercise and its role in cholesterol control. This chapter will focus on some other ways to help control your lipid levels.

OBTAINING AND MAINTAINING
IDEAL BODY WEIGHT

Several height and weight charts are available for use as gauges to help determine ideal body weight. The charts are typically based on your height, sex, and bone structure. Categories of small, medium, and large bone structures are the usual classifications listed. It is easy to determine into which category you fit. The bony diameter of your wrist is the place to determine your bone structure category. To make this measurement, circle your wrist with the thumb and index finger of your opposite hand. You should do this to yourself. Use the wrist of your dominant hand and the thumb and index finger of your nondominant hand. For example, if you are right-handed, place the thumb and index fingers of your left hand to encircle your right wrist. If your thumb and index finger do not meet, you have a large bone frame. If the thumb and index finger just meet, you have a medium frame. And finally, if they overlap, you fit the small frame category.

Ideal body weight is one of the determinations that will help you set a realistic weight goal. Your idea of ideal may be different from those prepared by the experts. Often your personal idea of what would be ideal is based on a fantasy, and undoubtedly colored by Madison Avenue's portrayal of model-thin. When using a chart to determine your ideal weight, notice that the weights are given in ranges. Practically speaking, everyone has fluctuations in weight. Keep in mind the ideal range is not one single number. Weight control must be practical and that means working within a range. The height and weight charts are frequently used because of their availability, but they do have drawbacks. They do not make a distinction between fat body weight and lean body weight. Because muscle, or lean mass, weighs more than fat mass, a person could be over their ideal body weight on the charts while maintaining very healthy and fit body composition. For this reason, it is probably more important to assess body composition rather than body weight alone.

Remember that while weight is certainly a concern, and being overweight is a significant potential health risk, especially in relation to heart disease, a more important consideration is body composition. A person may be well within his or her ideal body weight and still have too much fat. This is just one reason that analyzing body composition is more indicative of health and fitness. The terms overweight and obese are used frequently during discussions of weight and body composition. These two terms have clear definitions. Keeping in mind these definitions will help when discussing body weight. The term *overweight* refers to excess weight that is 10% more than ideal body weight. The term *obese* refers to a greater than 20% excess over the ideal weight. Body composition refers to the identification of the fat and nonfat elements that comprise weight. The body composition is made up of two parts: the fat mass and the lean mass. The fat mass is strictly measuring the fat stores and adipose tissue. Lean mass is primarily a measurement of muscle, bone, and connective tissue.

Within the fat mass compartment of the body, two distinctions are made. Essential body fat is the minimal amount of fat necessary for human function. In other words, it is essential to life. The essential body fat serves three basic functions: to insulate, to protect vital organs, and to assist in hormone regulation. Men require much less essential body fat than women. This is primarily due to hormone regulation and sex-specific fat like the breast tissue. Essential body fat for men is about 3% of total body weight. Essential body fat for women is about 12%. The second type of fat is the storage fat. Storage fat refers to the excess fat surrounding the organs and under the skin. Both men and women have storage fat. To determine the amount of fat mass and lean mass certain measurements must be accurately made and then calculations performed to determine the body composition. Several methods are used to determine body composition, including hydrostatic weighing, bioelectrical impedance, or anthropomorphic measurements commonly refered to as skin-fold assessment. All these methods require a degree of skill and equipment to evaluate body composition. It is not practical or easy to perform body composition testing on yourself in your home.

Because of the limitations of the height and weight charts and the complexity of the body composition tests, a relatively simple and yet accurate method for determining fat distribution was sought. In looking for a way to assess body composition, experts found that a major consideration was the distribution of fat stores. For instance, some people accumulate fat around the hips and thighs, while other tend to store excess fat around the waist and trunk. Those who store around the hips and thighs are said to be "pears." The people who store fat in the trunk and waist region are referred to as "apples." This seemed like a reasonable place to begin to look for a way to easily make the determination of body composition.

After several studies produced standards, it was determined that the ratio between the measurements of the hips and waist would be a simple at-home method of determining body fat distribution. Recent studies have shown that it is important to determine if you are a pear or an apple. Apples have a higher incidence of heart disease, hypertension, and diabetes.

To calculate the waist-to hip ratio, some very simple measurements are made to determine the amount of fat found in the hip region in relation to the amount found in the waist region.

Accurate measurements of both the waist and hip circumferences (distance around) are needed. To ensure accuracy, the following steps should be taken. First of all, dress with minimal or no clothing. Use a nonelastic tape measure and record the circumferences in inches. The circumference of the waist is measured at the most narrow point at the level of the belly button (umbilicus). The hips are measured at the largest point across the buttocks. Once the two measurements have been obtained, they can be expressed as a ratio using the following formula: Waist Circumference/Hip Circumference. This formula is fairly simple to use, as you will see in the example below.

If a person has a waist circumference of 42 inches and a hip circumference of 50 inches, you would divide 42/50, thereby giving the person a waist-to-hip ratio of 0.84. Generally speaking, the waist-to-hip ratio for men should be less than 0.95 and less than 0.85 for women. You can see how these simple measurements and calculations can easily help you determine your ideal body composition.

To help you obtain ideal body weight and fat distribution, you can use the strategies found in the remainder of this chapter. The same strategies that we will discuss for reaching your ideal weight and fat distribution can also be used for maintenance. The suggestions and ideas we recommend for weight and cholesterol control will work for a lifetime. This is not a "diet" that you go on and off, but rather a pleasant and practical approach to eating. To obtain and maintain ideal weight and fat distribution, it will be necessary for you to examine your eating habits. Eating is a habit, and analyzing it will show what areas of the habit you need to change for a healthier lifestyle. Most of the time we eat without thinking about it. It is this mindless eating that can cause you to overeat and become overweight. What follows are some suggestions that will give you greater control over eating, as well as add greater pleasure and satisfaction. After all, eating should be pleasurable. One sure way to increase the pleasure is to pay attention. This new level of awareness to your eating will help you with both your cholesterol control and weight control.

PAY ATTENTION TO YOUR BODY'S SIGNALS

We eat to give our body the nutrients and energy it needs. Food is fuel for the body. If we give the body too much fuel, it will store the additional food for future use. The body stores this excess fuel or food as fat. Fat is the body's means of storage. To obtain and maintain ideal body weight and composition, you must balance your intake of food with your output of energy. Your body will tell you when it needs nutrients and energy. Unfortunately, most of us have not been conditioned to pay attention to the signals that the body sends us. When your body needs food, you will get hungry. It is possible that some of you may have never experienced hunger. Hunger is different from appetite. Appetite is the *desire* for food, and hunger is the body's *need* for food. Because hunger is a physical need, the signals that you will get when you are hungry are physical. Some examples of hunger are a growling stomach, headache, loss of concentration, and irritability. Some examples of appetite are smelling fresh-baked bread, seeing a pie, watching T.V. commercials, or reading a restaurant menu. By these examples it is easy to tell hunger (physical needs), from appetite (desire). If you pay attention, you will be able to determine when you *need* to eat as opposed to when you *want* to eat. You will have to determine how your body "tells" you it is hungry, and then respond appropriately to those signals. You should learn to eat when you are hungry. To be more precise, you should eat only when you are optimally hungry. That sounds strange doesn't it? It isn't really; if you pay attention to your hunger signals you will be able to determine your degree of hunger.

One way to help you determine just how hungry you are is to use a rating system or scale. You can use a scale of one to five. A "one" means that you are hungry but can wait to eat; a "five" signifies that you are absolutely ravenous. If you wait for your hunger to get to a level five, you can see how it would be easy to overeat. This is usually done by eating a large amount of food in a short period of time. On the other hand, if you eat when your hunger is a level one, you probably won't eat enough and will want to eat again after a brief time has passed. You can see the dangers of eating at either end of the hunger scale. That is why we referred to optimal hunger, which for most of us is a level three or four on the hunger scale. Begin to eat when your hunger reaches a three or four in intensity, but that is not the end to controlling your eating. You must continue to rate your hunger through your meal. When you are no longer hungry, stop eating! This is an excellent way to begin to take control of your eating habits.

The second part of this strategy of eating appropriately is not only limiting your eating to when you are hungry, but to eating food that will satisfy you. You do this by eating food that tastes good to you. That sounds easy enough. In fact, some of you are probably thinking, what are they talking about? You may even be saying, "Of course I eat what tastes good to me." But to know if the food you are eating is good and will be satisfying, you must first taste it. How often do you really concentrate and taste your food?

Once again, try rating the taste of food on a scale of one to five. A "one" means you could take it or leave it, and a "five" means it is one of the most delicious things you have ever eaten. Once you have the rating scale in place, it will be easier to ask yourself, "Do I want to waste eating all of the extra calories and fat grams on a 'level one'?" The answer should be an emphatic no! Just as in the hunger scale you wanted to be in the middle range, so too do you want to eat mostly level "threes" and "fours" when rating taste. Most of your food choices should be "threes" and "fours," but don't deprive yourself of level "fives" now and then. We all need some "fives" in our lives! During the meal, continue to rate the taste of food because, as your hunger becomes satisfied, the taste of the food will diminish. When food falls to a "one" rating, it is time to stop eating.

If you use the hunger and taste-rating scales, you will begin to take control of your eating. Because you are eating only when you are hungry and stopping when your hunger is gone, you will find yourself beginning to lose some of that excess weight. Remember, when rating taste, you will actually prefer low-fat foods once you become accustomed to them. Give yourself a couple of months to develop a taste for foods that will be good to your heart. By doing this, you will find just how good they can taste.

Examining other eating habits will give you even more ways to obtain and maintain ideal body weight and composition. Ask yourself some questions related to your eating to help see which areas you may need to change. The questions are: When? Where? How frequently? and How long? The answers to these questions may not be as easy as you think. Once you examine your answers, they may be different than you thought they were on first glance. Let's take a look at these questions one at a time.

When do you eat? Do you always eat at certain times of the day? Or is eating automatically associated with particular activities? For instance, do you have meals at specific times every day regardless of what your energy output has been? Are snacks a necessary part of your T.V. viewing? Would a ball game be somehow incomplete without a hot dog and a beer? If you answered yes to any of these questions, or if they triggered you to come up with other examples of your own, then you are probably eating when you are not hungry. Remember you should eat because your body is sending you signals that it needs fuel. Instead you are eating in response to external stimulation—the time of day, the activity, or the company.

Where do you eat? If you are eating in front of the television, at your desk, or in your car, can you pay attention to the taste of the food and continually rate your taste and hunger? You should limit your eating to places that have been established for eating. These are called appropriate eating places. Some examples of appropriate eating places are the kitchen, dining room, cafeteria, restaurant, or picnic table. If you limit your eating to those appropriate, designated places, you will be surprised at how you will limit your food intake. Doing this will help you obtain or maintain ideal weight.

How frequently do you eat? Some of you eat virtually every waking hour of the day. Perhaps you are even one of those people who wake up from sleep to eat. Once again, this is habitual, mindless eating. If you eat in response to hunger, you will eliminate this continual type of overeating. Two additional considerations relate directly to the frequency of eating. First of all, do not eat after eight o'clock at night or four hours before going to bed. As we stated in the beginning of this section, food is fuel for the body. When your body is at rest, it uses much less fuel or energy. Therefore the food that you eat prior to sleep will not be needed as fuel. If it is not used, the body will store it. And, as you know, the body stores unused fuel as fat.

The second consideration is to emphasize the importance of eating breakfast. By eating in the morning, your body's metabolism wakes up. The sooner you increase metabolism the sooner you will begin burning more fuel. All of you expert dieters know that if you don't eat breakfast, you can sometimes go until noon without feeling hungry. But if you eat breakfast you actually start to feel hungry earlier. This is a good thing! Hunger means that your body has used fuel and needs more. This shows that your body is working at a higher metabolic rate. So don't skip a delicious low-fat breakfast; start burning up those calories.

How long are your meals? Just as important as the factors we have examined above is how long a meal lasts. The optimal time for a meal is 20–25 minutes. This time factor is not a suggestion, but rather the result of scientific research. It takes 20–25 minutes for the stomach to send a signal to the brain, and then for the brain to respond to the fact that the stomach is full. If you eat too quickly, your brain may not receive its signal from the stomach, and consequently you will soon be hungry again. On the other hand, if you take too long to eat, your appetite center in the brain can be restimulated, causing you to overeat. Look at the clock before you begin a meal and try to keep eating time in the twenty-minute range. If you are outside the twenty-minute range, either too long or too short, you will have to take measures to correct your eating habits.

If you eat too quickly, you will need to prolong your eating time. Since eating more is probably not the objective, you will have to learn other ways to do this. You can use utensils and frequently put them down. Using a napkin to wipe your mouth between bites is another helpful technique. Cutting food into small bite-size pieces will also aid in prolonging meal-time. One method that can be used to help you identify ways to slow your eating is to actually eat in front of a mirror. Remember as you watch yourself in the mirror that this is the way others see you when you eat.

Those of you on the other end of the time scale may need to speed up your meal to fit within the twenty-minute optimal time. You may need to take smaller portions, or limit conversation during a meal. Pay attention to your food, enjoy it, taste it, and rate your hunger during the meal. All of these strategies will help keep your meal in the proper time frame.

If you begin to correct your inappropriate eating habits, you will find that you can lose weight to obtain your ideal body weight and composition. Be patient. Changing habits takes time. You didn't develop your eating behaviors overnight, and you won't be able to change them that quickly either. When you conquer a new eating behavior, encourage yourself with a reward. The rewards should be nonfood, such as playing a new CD, reading a book, buying clothes, taking a long bath, going for a walk, or talking with a friend. The reward can be anything special that says you've done a good job! To succeed in changing eating habits, it's important to have patience and give yourself rewards.

LIMITING CHOLESTEROL WILL
HELP CONTROL BLOOD LIPIDS

As you have read in the previous chapters, limiting your intake of cholesterol will help control your blood lipids. Remember that cholesterol is found in foods from animal sources. Especially high concentrations of cholesterol are contained in the organ meats of animals and in the skin of fowl. Therefore, it is very important that your intake of these foods be limited. The recommendation is that cholesterol intake be limited to less than 300 mg per day. If a person is restricting cholesterol to the recommendation of less than 300 mg a day and is carefully controlling fat intake to meet the less than 30% total daily calorie intake (with saturated fat restricted to less than 10%), but has still not obtained a blood cholesterol of 200 mg/dL, further action must be taken.

The restrictions listed above and in Chapter 5 are consistent with the American Heart Association Step I diet. A Step II diet may be necessary if the blood cholesterol does not reach the acceptable range on Step I. The Step II diet further limits the intake of cholesterol to less than 200 mg a day. The Step II diet additionally restricts saturated fats to less than 7% of total daily calories. It is important to remember that limiting cholesterol is only one step in the process to lower blood cholesterol. Several other measures are necessary, in combination with the restriction of cholesterol intake, to succeed in lowering the blood cholesterol to the recommended range. If you follow cholesterol and fat intake restrictions, as well as maintain an ideal body weight and composition, exercise regularly, stop smoking, and adhere to any medication program that your physician may prescribe, you will be doing your best to fight elevated cholesterol and heart disease.

STOP SMOKING—NOW!!!!

Smoking is one of the major contributors to cardio-vascular disease and heart attack. In addition, smoking is the major cause of lung disease and cancers. The effects of smoking are cumulative. That means if you have never smoked, you are better off than someone who has smoked for a year and then stopped. If you have smoked for ten years, you have more damage than someone who smoked for five, but less than someone who has smoked for twenty. To be even more practical, if you quit smoking today, you will have less damage than if you quit tomorrow. Smoking does have an effect on the blood cholesterol and triglyceride levels. Smokers have lower HDL (good) cholesterol and higher levels of LDL (bad) cholesterol. If you want to do everything you can to help reduce your risk of heart disease, you will stop smoking now in addition to following the other recommendations in this book.

Stopping smoking isn't easy, *but it can be done!* There are now more ex-smokers in the United States than there are smokers. Studies have shown that smoking in the United States has declined by 32% since 1965. That's the good news, but there are still a large number of smokers. It is currently estimated that 24.2 million men smoke. That is 28.4% of the male pop-ulation. Of the female population, 21.6 million women smoke. This represents 22.8% of the female population. The distressing news is that 2.4 million teenagers between the ages of 12 and 17 smoke. The Center of Disease Control (CDC) estimates that every day 3,000 American youngsters become smokers. Statistically, 75% of adult smokers started before age 18 and 90% began before age 21. Frequently young people say they will experiment with smoking, but know that it can cause health problems so they will stop before that happens to them. We can see from the numbers reported by the CDC that this is not the case.

Recent studies have shown that women who smoke and use oral contraceptives are at increased risk for heart attack and stroke. Just how great are these risks? Women who smoke and use oral contraceptives are 39 times more likely to suffer a heart attack and 22 times more likely to suffer a stroke than women who neither smoke nor use oral birth control.

There has been much discussion and debate in the last several years with regard to secondhand smoke. The American Heart Association reports that in 1988 about 430,000 adults age 35 and older died of voluntary cigarette smoking, and 201,000 of these deaths were from cardiovascular causes. It is further reported that about 37,000 *nonsmokers* died of cardiovascular disease from having been exposed to environmental tobacco smoke (secondhand smoke).

If you do not smoke don't start. Furthermore, do everything you can to discourage youngsters from ever starting. As we have stated, stopping smoking is not easy, but don't give up on yourself. It is never too late to give up a bad habit. About 70% of all ex-smokers failed at least once before successfully quitting. From analyzing the literature, it appears that those who quit "cold turkey" have a higher success rate than those who "taper off." To be a successful ex-smoker, you may need help. Don't be afraid to find a program or an individual who may be able to help you. It is important to know why you smoke. Does it relax you? Try substituting deep breathing and relaxation exercises while you are stopping. Do you like the taste? If so, you may want to substitute mints, gum, or hard candy for that taste sensation you think you will be missing. Or are you the type of individual that needs to keep your hands busy? Replace that cigarette with a paper clip, a rubber band, an exercise ball, or marbles like Captain Queeg. When trying to stop smoking, it is helpful to go places where smoking is prohibited. This has become easier in many states with new laws that restrict smoking in public places. Finally, watch ex-smokers and nonsmokers. See what they are doing and imitate their behavior. Talk to ex-smokers and find out what helped them; it just may help you too. Put down those cigarettes right now and help raise your overall health!

FOLLOW YOUR DOCTOR'S ADVICE

The best and first treatment choice for lowering cholesterol is always diet, but sometimes diet alone can't sufficiently reduce the cholesterol. In those cases, drug therapy will be added. Medications are *never* a substitute for diet. In fact, a diet that is high in saturated fats and cholesterol can actually minimize the effects of drug therapy. When your physician prescribes a cholesterol-lowering medication, it is out of necessity. Medication in combination with a low-fat, low-cholesterol diet is yet another way to help win the war with cholesterol. Medications used in lowering cholesterol levels will be discussed in Chapter 13.

To help control cholesterol, you should obtain and maintain ideal body weight and composition, stop smoking, establish a regular exercise program, and take any lipid-lowering medications that have been prescribed for you. All of these steps must be done in conjunction with following the low-fat, low-cholesterol diet recommendations. By following all of these suggestions, you can control your cholesterol.

Cholesterol is a killer, so you must be ready to fight back in as many ways as you can. A well-rounded lifestyle that incorporates all of the cholesterol-lowering suggestions will help you have a longer and healthier life.

11

Women and Heart Disease

Despite significant improvements in diagnosis and care of heart problems, cardiovascular disease is still the number one cause of death in the United States. Contrary to popular perception, cardiovascular disease affects both men and women. The unmistakable point must be made that heart disease is the number one killer of women in the United States. More women die of heart disease than from all forms of cancer combined. Significant years of productive life are lost because of premature death due to coronary heart disease.

As you have read, a low HDL cholesterol and a high LDL cholesterol level have both been well established as powerful risk factors for the development of coronary heart disease. You should remember that the "well established risk factors" are based on large studies made up almost exclusively of men. Only in recent years have studies begun to focus on women and heart disease because there was an obvious lack of specific information available. For women, several independent studies have shown HDL cholesterol and triglyceride levels were the best predictors of heart disease. These studies found that, in addition to the recognized risk factors for Coronary Heart Disease (CHD), the following risks were identified as particular to women: diabetes, hormonal status, use of oral contraceptives and cigarettes together, and level of education. We would like to take a closer look at these "female factors" since they create an additional risk for women beyond the traditional risk factors discussed earlier in the book.

HORMONAL STATUS

First, the hormonal status of women has a great influence on the development of atherosclerosis and subsequent formation of coronary heart disease. Premenopausal women are somewhat protected against coronary heart disease. Between the ages of 45 and 64, women suffer about one-third the number of heart attacks that occur in men of the same age. After age 65, the incidence of coronary heart disease in women increases and is close to the same incidence for men ages 45–64. While it is true that women develop coronary heart disease about ten years later in life than men, the death rate for these women is much higher than for the men.

In premenopausal women, the HDL cholesterol is usually greater than in postmenopausal women. As we have already discussed, increased levels of HDL are protective against heart disease. While it is true that premenopausal women have generally higher HDL levels, their LDL levels vary during the menstrual cycle. Studies have shown as much as a 10–25% variation in women's cholesterol levels throughout the menstrual cycle. This is due to the fact that the body increases its fat storage in preparation for pregnancy. Increased fats are necessary during pregnancy and during lactation. In most women these elevations are temporary and return to their baseline following the cessation of lactation or if the woman does not nurse after delivery. The elevation in LDL cholesterol during pregnancy and lactation are thought to be a normal event, and studies have shown that this temporary elevation does not have a detrimental effect on the cardiovascular system.

Not only is this hormonal influence seen in pre- and post menopausal women, but it is also present in those taking hormone replacement medications (estrogen or progestin). In reproductive-aged women taking oral contraceptives, there have been proven differences in their lipid profiles based on whether it is an estrogen-dominant or progestin-dominant oral contraceptive medication. Those taking estrogen-dominant oral contraceptives had LDL levels that were unchanged and HDL levels that were increased. The women taking progestin-dominant oral contraceptives had a significant increase in their LDL and a decrease in their HDL cholesterol levels. It makes sense that, since estrogen raises HDL cholesterol without increasing LDL cholesterol, estrogen would have a protective effect against coronary heart disease. Whether the estrogen is intrinsic (produced by the ovaries in premenopausal women) or extrin-sic (taken in pill or shot form from outside the body) does not seem to matter. Studies show that postmenopausal women who receive estrogen replacements decrease their cardiovascular disease risk by 30–70%.

If this is true, then why don't all women take estrogen replacement once they reach menopause? As in all things, estrogen does not affect cholesterol levels alone. Thus, there is the potential for other significant non-cholesterol adverse effects on the body. In light of this information, it is important that women carefully discuss treatment options with their physician.

DIABETES

Diabetes has been shown to be more of a risk for women in the development of coronary heart disease than for men. Diabetes is a risk for both men and women, but when factored out, it represents a greater independent risk for women than men. This may be due to the increase in triglycerides that usually accompany diabetes. This triglyceride increase was more impressive in diabetic women than in diabetic men. Both diabetes and elevated triglycerides are independent risks in women.

CIGARETTES AND ORAL CONTRACEPTIVES

The combined use of cigarettes and oral contraceptives causes increased risk of cardiovascular disease (see Chapter 10). The combined use is worse than cigarette smoking alone. For this reason, women who use oral contraceptives are strongly discouraged from smoking cigarettes.

EDUCATIONAL STATUS

The final risk particular to women is a low educational status. The significance of this has been hotly debated, but no one single reason for this risk can be found. It is probably a combination of factors that account for the increased cardiovascular risk associated with educational status. Perhaps difficulty with label reading and the inability to make wise food choices may account for part of the increased risk. Additionally, awareness of heart disease in general and as a health concern for women in particular may encourage women to seek medical help earlier than someone less educated. We do not attempt to fully explain this finding but rather present it to encourage women to be aware of all aspects of their health and to do their part to take responsibility.

Now that the lack of information related to women and heart disease has been recognized, several large studies are presently being conducted to research these facts. As with cholesterol information in general, as time goes on, our knowledge should increase. This increased knowledge should help decrease the incidence of coronary heart disease in the future. Despite making significant advances in knowledge, education, and treatment in the last decade, cardiovascular disease still remains the number one cause of death in men and women.

12 Kids and Cardiovascular Disease

If the current rate of heart disease does not change, two of every four children will develop cardiovascular disease as an adult and one of those two children will die from a heart attack as an adult. It is one thing to discuss the risk of cardiovascular disease and the fact that it causes one of every two deaths in the United States, but the importance of these numbers and this disease takes on new meaning when relating it to children. Would any parent want his or her child to be the one with cardiovascular disease? Since cardiovascular disease can be prevented or decreased by risk factor management, it would make sense for parents to take responsibility for teaching their children healthy habits that will last a lifetime.

Presently, half of all children ages 7–12 have elevated blood cholesterol levels and 28% of this age group have hypertension. The story gets worse, as 13% of all children ages 2–18 are overweight. This overweight problem is one that is fairly new. Since 1960, childhood obesity has risen 54% and super-obesity has risen 98%. As you have learned, high cholesterol levels, high blood pressure, and obesity are all risk factors for the development of heart disease. You also have learned that the more risk factors you accumulate, the greater your chance of actually developing cardiovascular disease. Currently 98% of American children have at least one risk factor, and 67% have three or more factors. It is critical for the health of the nation's children that these risks be brought under control. All children should have their cholesterol checked by the time they reach school age. It is even more important that children with a family history of heart disease or elevated cholesterol, or any additional risk factors, have their cholesterol level checked.

ELEVATED CHOLESTEROL IN CHILDREN

The previous chapters of this book have tried to give you a clear explanation of how elevated blood cholesterol levels contribute to the development of cardiovascular disease including heart attack, stroke, high blood pressure, and aneurysm formation. While there is certainly a familial factor to elevated blood cholesterol, in many cases dietary management is all that is necessary to control the elevated cholesterol. And even in instances when drug therapy is needed, dietary control remains the primary key to regulating the blood cholesterol. For this reason it is important to teach children how to make wise low-fat food choices. The reason many Americans have elevated cholesterol is not because elevated cholesterol is inherited, but rather because they learned to eat at their parents' table. Eating is a habit. Adult eating habits are usually learned during childhood and continued through life.

It is vitally important to teach children about cholesterol, and how to control it with good low-fat food choices. Think about it: The number one way to die in the United States is from heart disease. We know that elevated cholesterol leads to heart disease. Since cholesterol levels can be controlled through wise eating, wouldn't it be sensible to teach your children how to reduce the risk of cardiovascular disease, the number one killer in this country? We teach our children to obey traffic laws, buckle their seat belts, not talk to strangers, and a million other things to keep them safe and healthy. How can we continue to teach them, by example, how to eat high-fat foods that will kill them? Isn't this like showing them how to ingest poison? Remember that the American Heart Association Step I low-fat, low-cholesterol diet is recommended for *everyone over the age of two.*

Children under two years of age *should not* have their fat intake restricted. High fat is absolutely necessary for development and growth during the first two years. But after age two, a Step I diet is recommended. Children should be taught about saturated and unsaturated fats and how to identify them. If children are introduced to this type of thinking, they will make low-fat choices. Remember, eating is a habit, so it is very important for you to set a good example for children.

It is sad to report that over 80% of children between the ages of two and five consume more total fat, saturated fat, and cholesterol than is recommended. This increased intake of fat over a lifetime is one cause of atherosclerosis. The formation of blockages in the arteries does not happen over one or two months or even one or two years, but rather over a lifetime of consuming a high-fat diet. It is easy to see how the 80% of children with high-fat diets will become the same people who develop heart disease. Studies have repeatedly proven that the beginning signs of atherosclerosis are found in children over the age of nine in this country. Isn't it alarming that by age nine, children are already showing signs of a disease that may cause them health problems or cost them their lives? This reinforces the need to start young in teaching children how to identify saturated fat and how to read food labels when they are old enough to do so.

Many studies have been done with regard to school lunch programs and the Step I guidelines. In general, the average lunch selected by students has 35% of its calories from fat. As you can see, this is above the recommended 30% or less. Additionally, in the lunches selected by children, 12.6% of the calories were from saturated fat. Once again, this is outside the less than 10% guideline for saturated fat calories.

You may think that these results are because children want to eat or prefer a high-fat diet and would not eat low-fat choices even if they were available. But if we look further at these school lunch studies, we find that when given the choice of low-fat foods, more than a third of the children choose to eat the low-fat meal over the high-fat alternative. Since very little cholesterol education is given to children, consider the impact a cholesterol education program could have. It is important to point out that we acquire tastes and that those tastes or likes and dislikes are a result of habit. In persons changing to a low-fat diet, most found high-fat foods unpleasant to the taste after two to three months. This is good news for both you and your children. If the family begins a low-fat diet, it will become second nature in a few short months to the point that everyone will prefer the taste of low-fat foods.

CHILDREN AND EXERCISE

The youth of today are much less physically active than children of even ten years ago. This is due to a multitude of factors. The result, regardless of the cause, is that we have a society in which children are increasingly overweight, less fit, and at higher risk for cardiovascular disease. Studies show that the health benefits from an active lifestyle are many and varied, age notwithstanding. Children must be encouraged and taught by example to engage in regular physical activities. In a study done of middle-school-aged children, the dominant factor in whether the child participated in routine physical activity was whether the parent exercised regularly. This was true of both boys and girls. The fact that adult exercise encourages children to do likewise should be yet another incentive for American adults to get up and exercise.

Unfortunately, children do not currently have good role models in this respect. In a National Health Interview, 24% of the adult population reported no routine physical activity. Approximately one in ten Americans report thirty minutes of daily physical activity. In fact only 7.6% of the population of the United States exercises at levels recommended to achieve cardiovascular benefits.

The National Children and Youth Fitness Study reported that at least half of all children do not engage in physical activity that would be conducive to promoting good health. The same study also reported that less than 36% of the schools, both elementary and secondary, offer daily physical education classes. And of the physical education hours offered, minimal time was spent doing activities that were likely to nurture lifelong physical activity and fitness habits.

Physical activity reduces the risk of developing cardiovascular disease and helps regulate high blood pressure and diabetes. Additionally, physical activity helps combat overweight by promoting weight loss, while maintaining or increasing lean body mass. All people who are physically active are less likely to smoke than their sedentary counterparts, including adolescents and teenagers. Routine physical activity is one of the cornerstones in the prevention of heart disease, and it should start in childhood.

The children of today will be better able to prevent heart disease from remaining the number one killer in their generation if adults set good examples for them in cardiovascular health.

13 When Diet Alone Isn't Enough

Unfortunately, following the dietary recommendations of a low-fat and low-cholesterol diet may not be enough for some people to sufficiently reduce their cholesterol to an acceptable range. Those individuals may require prescription lipid-lowering medications. When medication is required, it is *always in addition to dietary control*. It has been shown that the beneficial effect of the medications can be significantly reduced if a person continues to eat a diet high in cholesterol and saturated fats. For this reason, it is important to continue with the kind of dietary changes that are found in this book and coincide with the recommendations of the American Heart Association.

If medication is necessary, what kind of drug therapy should be prescribed? Traditionally, the medication used for cholesterol-lowering purposes is a type of medicine called a bile acid sequestrant. However, several other medicines can be used and in fact are used more commonly now. These other medications include niacin (nicotinic acid), Lopid (gemfibrozil), and HMG CoA reductase Inhibitors (Mevacor, Zocor, Pravacol, and Lescol). Each medication will be discussed in turn.

BILE ACID SEQUESTRANTS

Two medications in the bile acid sequestrant category have the trade names Questran and Colestid. These powders work in the intestinal tract and are not absorbed by the body. Questran and Colestid trap cholesterol in the intestine like a sponge soaking up water. They "hold" the cholesterol and eliminate it from the body in the stool. These medications lower total cholesterol and LDL cholesterol, but they do not reduce triglyceride levels and actually may cause a rise in triglycerides. Bile acid sequestrants also may raise HDL cholesterol 3–8%. Total cholesterol is lowered about 10% and LDL cholesterol can be lowered as much as 10–20%. General experience indicates the improvements in cholesterol tend to occur more frequently near the lower range of improvement. In the Lipid Research Clinics Coronary Primary Prevention Trial (LRC CPPT), Questran was used by the men who did not receive a placebo. The LRC CPPT showed that the 9% reduction in the total cholesterol resulted in a 19% reduction in the incidence of coronary heart disease.

What are the side effects of this type of medicine? The bile acid sequestrants are safe medications; however, they do have some side effects that people find uncomfortable and/or unpleasant. Because Questran and Colestid work in the intestinal tract and are excreted in the stool, the most common side effects are associated with gastrointestinal discomfort. Bloating, indigestion, gas, and constipation are the most common side effects. These side effects occur because bile, which contains the cholesterol in the intestine, is trapped by the medications and is then eliminated in the stool. Bile is a digestive aid and is an irritant to the bowel. Adding fruits, vegetables, and high fiber grains to the diet will help reduce or eliminate these gastrointestinal side effects.

In addition to the gastrointestinal side effects, Questran and Colestid trap and eliminate some medications that you may be taking. Therefore, Questran and Colestid should *not* be taken on the same time schedule as other medications. It is generally recommended that other medications be taken at least one hour before, or four to six hours after taking the Questran or Colestid. Ask your doctor about how to most effectively take all of your medications. As with all medicines, these should not be stopped abruptly without your physician's knowlege and approval.

NIACIN (NICOTINIC ACID)

Nicotinic acid, or niacin, can be used alone or in combination with the other cholesterol-lowering medicines. Nicotinic acid is a B vitamin. In doses that are far larger than those needed as a vitamin, nicotinic acid usually lowers total cholesterol, LDL cholesterol, and triglycerides. Nicotinic acid also tends to raise the HDL (good) cholesterol. These effects can be seen with doses of 1.5 grams (1,500 milligrams) per day, but doses as high as 6 grams (6,000 milligrams) may be required to get the desired effect. Usually doses of less than 1.5 grams per day have little beneficial effect on the blood cholesterol levels. Nicotinic acid comes in 100, 250, and 500 mg (milligram) tablets. As you would imagine, the 500 mg tablets are the most practical because of the amount of nicotinic acid that needs to be taken daily to get a beneficial cholesterol effect. The niacin should be rapid release (not slow release) as will be explained later, and should be taken with meals to lessen the side effects. Even though niacin (nicotinic acid) is non-prescription and can be bought over the counter in a pharmacy or health food store, it must be considered a medicine when used in large doses and should only be used under the guidance and monitoring of a physician.

What are the side effects of niacin? Flushing is the most common side effect of niacin. Flushing usually occurs about 30 to 60 minutes after taking a dose of rapid-release niacin. It is characterized by a warm feeling, usually in the face and ears, accompanied by redness. It is not painful, but is considered an unpleasant feeling. The "flush" usually lasts for about 30 minutes or less. It does not always occur after a dose of niacin and can be blocked by taking an aspirin about 30 minutes before the niacin dose. Also, taking the niacin at mealtime tends to reduce the side effects and flushing. Itching can accompany the flushing or can occur by itself. The itching is usually minor, but occasionaly it is extremely annoying and requires stopping the niacin. The itching is also blocked by taking an aspirin before the niacin dose. To get around the itching and flushing side effects, a slow-release niacin was developed. However, niacin can also cause inflammation in the liver, which rarely leads to significant liver damage. Episodes in which significant liver problems occurred, however, were limited almost totally to slow-release niacin use. For this reason, slow-release niacin should not be used for cholesterol control. Niacin can also cause problems in people with a previous history of stomach problems or ulcers, raise blood sugar in diabetics, increase uric acid levels in the blood and cause gout, cause skin rashes, and, rarely, cause problems with the heart rhythm. Despite this apparently long list of side effects, niacin is an excellent medicine for controlling cholesterol. It can be used alone or in combination with some of the other cholesterol medicines. Again, niacin should only be used under the direction and guidance of a physician, who will also monitor the cholesterol levels and liver enzyme blood tests.

LOPID (GEMFIBROZIL)

Lopid (gemfibrozil) belongs to a type of lipid-lowering drug family called fibrates. Exactly how lopid works is really not understood. Lopid is very useful in lowering triglyceride levels and raising HDL cholesterol levels. Additionally, Lopid also tends to lower total cholesterol and LDL cholesterol. The effects on total and LDL cholesterol tend to be less dramatic than gemfibrozil's effects on triglycerides and HDL cholesterol levels. Lopid can occasionally cause an increase in LDL cholesterol as well. The Helsinki Study compared the use of Lopid to a placebo in 4,081 men. The results showed the total cholesterol and LDL cholesterol were both lowered 8%. Triglycerides were reduced by 35%, and HDL cholesterol increased by 10%. The end result was that the group of men taking Lopid had a 34% reduction in coronary heart disease when compared to the group taking the placebo. This study suggests that raising HDL cholesterol in addition to lowering LDL cholesterol and triglycerides is beneficial. The usual dose of Lopid is 600 mg twice a day.

What are the side effects of Lopid? Lopid does not have many side effects. Most people can tolerate this medicine without difficulty. The incidence of nausea and diarrhea, which are the primary side effects, are low. Lopid can sometimes promote or accelerate the formation of gallstones.

THE NEWEST FAMILY OF MEDICINES IN THE FIGHT AGAINST CHOLESTEROL

HMG CoA reductase Inhibitors are a new family of medications that dramatically lower the blood cholesterol and LDL cholesterol levels. These have been in use for about a decade. Lovastatin (Mevacor) was the original member of the family approved for use in the U.S. in 1987, but there are now three other related medicines used to lower the cholesterol levels. These include pravastatin (Pravacol), simvastatin (Zocor), and fluvastatin (Lescol).

In Chapter 2, you learned that the body can make cholesterol, which is necessary for certain essential bodily functions. The primary production site for this endogenous cholesterol is the liver. The liver makes about 70% of all the cholesterol produced by the body. This production is how your body guarantees that it will always have enough cholesterol. Lovastatin and its family members block the production of cholesterol in the liver by stopping the action of a necessary enzyme. When the liver is prohibited from making cholesterol, absorption of cholesterol from the blood is increased to meet the body's demands. The liver increases its absorption of cholesterol from the blood by increasing the number of places that LDL cholesterol can be received into the liver. Since the liver is removing LDL cholesterol from the blood, there is less LDL cholesterol left in the blood. In various studies, the family of HMG CoA reductase Inhibitors reduce blood LDL cholesterol by about 30–40%, and total cholesterol by 30–35%. In addition, triglycerides may decrease by

10–30%, and HDL cholesterol has a tendency to increase 2–15%. HMG CoA reductase Inhibitors do a remarkable job of lowering LDL and total cholesterol levels. Unlike some of the other cholesterol-lowering medications, they do not seem to interfere with other medications taken at the same time.

The HMG CoA reductase Inhibitors should generally be taken with the evening meal, as cholesterol production in the liver is greatest in the evening. The effects of the HMG CoA reductase Inhibitors on the blood cholesterol levels are related to the different dosage levels of the various medications. The greatest cholesterol lowering is acheived with the lowest dose, and there is an increased but less strong effect as the dosage level is raised. It should also be noted that each individual may respond to the medicines differently. The reduction numbers given above are an average and may be higher or lower for individuals.

The HMG CoA reductase Inhibitors are exciting medicines that can be used to help control cholesterol. However, some precautions must be considered. With the development of these very effective medicines that can lower LDL cholesterol as much as 40%, many people think they can "just take a pill" and cure their cholesterol problems. This simply isn't true. This medication, like all the others we have discussed, must be used in combination with a low-cholesterol and low-fat diet to be effective. Since cholesterol control must be for a lifetime, it is very important to follow a low-cholesterol, low-saturated-fat diet rather than depend on a medication alone. The HMG CoA reductase Inhibitors, like the majority of the cholesterol-lowering medicines, are expensive. Their longtime use can place a significant financial burden on the user. This is another reason to try to control cholesterol with diet alone or diet with minimal amounts of medications.

The HMG CoA reductase Inhibitors are extremely effective medicines but have not been used as long as other medications for cholesterol control. The long-term history of the drugs and their side effects are not currently available because of this. All medications have side effects as well as beneficial effects, and the HMG CoA reductase Inhibitors are no exception. This family of drugs has minor side effects of headache, nausea, insomnia, fatigue, muscle aches, and skin rashes. Less common but more important side effects include elevations in liver enzymes and myopathy (inflammation of the muscles). Increases in liver enzymes are dose dependent, and increases of enzyme levels to greater than three times normal occur in about 0.5–2% of people taking the medicine. In the majority of people, there are no symptoms related to the elevation of liver enzymes. Stopping the medicine or reducing the dose will usually return the liver enzyme levels to normal without any harm occurring.

To monitor patients on HMG CoA reductase Inhibitors, it is recommended that blood be checked every two to three months initially for the first six to twelve months and then every three to four months after that. Myopathy causes aching pain in the muscles and is associated with elevation of muscle enzymes. Myopathy occurs rarely (in about 1 out of 1,000 people) when the HMG CoA reductase Inhibitors are used by themselves. The incidence of myopathy increases when the HMG CoA reductase Inhibitors are used with Lopid (gemfibrozil), erythromycin (an antibiotic), niacin (nicotinic acid), and pronestyl (a heart rhythm drug). Even in combination, the occurrence of myopathy is rare. Stopping the medicines should reverse the effect on the muscles. When lovastatin (Mevacor) was first released, it was thought that it may cause opacifications in the lens of the eye. Because of this, it was originally recommended that users of lovastatin have a yearly eye exam. Large studies have shown that this belief was wrong and that lovastatin does not increase the chance of eye lens opacifications.

WHICH IS THE RIGHT MEDICINE FOR ME?

With several different medicines available to lower cholesterol, which is the best one for your doctor to start you on? There is no correct answer for this question. If you would see three different physicians, there is a good chance all three would treat your elevated cholesterol differently. There isn't necessarily a right and wrong way to treat the cholesterol. In fact, many different ways may end up at the same result.

When the total blood cholesterol and LDL cholesterol are elevated and meet the recommendations for treating with a medication in addition to diet, the official recommendation is to use a bile acid sequestrant first. However, in reality, this is rarely done. The two main reasons for skipping this medicine are because of the gastrointestinal side effects that many people have and the relatively small effect the bile acid sequestrant has on the blood cholesterol level. The most commonly prescribed medicine usually will be in the HMG CoA reductase Inhibitor family. Another alternative is to use niacin (nicotinic acid) as a first-line medication. Again, medication is always used in addition to a low-cholesterol, low-saturated-fat diet.

When the triglycerides are elevated without significant elevation of the LDL cholesterol, then Lopid (gemfibrozil) will usually be the first-line medication. Niacin (nicotinic acid) is also effective in lowering the blood triglyceride level. In patients with severe elevation of the triglycerides (>1,000), fish oil can also be beneficial in lowering the triglycerides. Fish oil is generally added to Lopid (gemfibrozil) and/or niacin therapy in these cases. Currently, there is significant debate about using a medication to raise an abnormally low HDL cholesterol. If the indications for trying to raise the HDL cholesterol level are met (see Chapter 2), generally Lopid (gemfibrozil), niacin (nicotinic acid), or a combination of the two are the most effective medications.

WHEN ONE MEDICINE IS NOT ENOUGH

In some people, a low-cholesterol, low-saturated-fat diet and one medication still does not bring the blood cholesterol levels into acceptable ranges. In these cases, two medications may be added together. The beneficial cholesterol effects of all of these medicines are additive. This means that cholesterol effects of the two medicines should be better than any one of the medicines alone. Caution should be exercised, though, because the adverse or side effects also can be additive and occur more frequently. The more commonly used combinations of medicines include an HMG CoA reductase Inhibitor and a bile acid sequestrant, or niacin and a bile acid sequestrant. Niacin and an HMG CoA reductase Inhibitor can be very effective but elevation of liver enzymes needs to be carefully monitored. Rarely, an HMG CoA reductase Inhibitor and Lopid (gemfibrozil) are used together. This is potentially a dangerous combination because of the increased problems with myopathy. Any person taking a cholesterol-lowering medication, and especially a combination of medicines, needs to be carefully monitored by a physician. You should contact your doctor promptly if you are taking any of these medicines or combinations and you have a problem.

ADDITIONAL INFORMATION

The last part of this chapter is optional reading. The information that follows represents the recommendations of the expert panel of the National Cholesterol Education Program. The first recommendations were issued in 1987 and have undergone minor modifications in 1993. This information is available to all physicians. These guidelines have been simplified in this chapter to make them more understandable. They are presented so that you know what the experts have recommended concerning detection and treatment of hyperlipidemia.

1987 RECOMMENDATIONS OF THE NCEP WITH 1993 UPDATED RECOMMENDATIONS OF THE NCEP II

The 1987 report of the National Cholesterol Education Program Expert Panel on Detection, Evaluation, and Treatment of High Blood Cholesterol in Adults (NCEP) made specific recommendations to all physicians concerning evaluation and treatment of blood cholesterol levels. The recommendations were reviewed and updated in 1993 by the NCEP Adult Treatment Panel II. These recommendations are presented here in written form and in Appendix 1 in flowchart form. Reading the written explanation and then referring to the flowchart will make understanding the recommendations easier. In addition, the flowchart will be easier to refer to for future reference once the information below is read and understood. These guidelines, from this panel of national experts, are available to all physicians in the United States.

Initial Classification

- Every adult age twenty and over should have a non-fasting total blood cholesterol level test, and HDL cholesterol should be measured at the same time if accurate results are available.
- All blood cholesterol levels above 200 mg/dL should be repeated, and the average used to guide clinical decisions.
- Coronary Heart Disease (CHD) risk factors as defined in this report include:

Positive risk factors:

- Age greater or equal to 45 in men or age greater than or equal to 55 in women or premature menopause without estrogen replacement therapy
- Family history of heart attack or sudden death before age 55 in a parent or brother or sister
- Cigarette smoking (currently smoke more than 0 cigarettes per day)
- High blood pressure
- HDL cholesterol less than 35 mg/dL
- Diabetes

Negative Risk Factors:

- HDL cholesterol greater than or equal to 60 mg/dL

Primary Prevention in Adults Without
Evidence of Coronary Heart Disease (CHD)

- All patients with a total cholesterol level of 240 mg/dL or higher should have a fasting lipid profile performed.
- Patients with a total cholesterol level of 200–239 mg/dL and two CHD risk factors or HDL cholesterol less than 35 should have a fasting lipid profile performed.
- Patients with a total cholesterol level of less than 200 and HDL cholesterol less than 35 should have a fasting lipid profile performed.
- Patients with a total cholesterol level of less than 200 and HDL cholesterol greater than or equal to 35 should have repeat total cholesterol and HDL cholesterol measurement within five years or with a physical exam.
- Patients with a total cholesterol level of 200–239 mg/dL and no CHD and one or less CHD risk factors and HDL cholesterol greater than 34 should be provided with information on dietary modification, physical activity, and risk factor reduction. They should be reevaluated in one to two years with repeat total and HDL cholesterol measurements.

Classification Based on LDL Cholesterol

If a fasting lipid profile was recommended above, dietary or drug therapy is decided on the LDL cholesterol levels. A fasting specimen should be at least a 12-hour fast with total cholesterol, HDL cholesterol, and triglycerides measured. An average of two measurements over one to eight weeks should be made for decision-making purposes.

- If LDL level is less than 130 mg/dL, general dietary and risk factor education should be given and total cholesterol and HDL cholesterol remeasured within five years.
- If LDL level is 130–159 mg/dL with one or less CHD risk factors, then patients should adhere to Step I AHA diet and recheck total cholesterol annually.
- If LDL level is greater than or equal to 160 mg/dL or 130–159 mg/dL with two or more CHD risk factors, patient should have clinical evaluation and LDL goal set. The LDL goal is less than 160 mg/dL or less than 130 mg/dL when two or more CHD risk factors are present.

Secondary Prevention in Adults With
Evidence of Coronary Heart Disease (CHD)
or Other Atherosclerotic Disease

Fasting lipid profile is required in all adults with known coronary artery disease, carotid artery disease, or peripheral vascular disease. Classification is then based on LDL cholesterol.

- For these patients, optimal LDL levels are 100 mg/dL or less.
- If the LDL is 100 mg/dL or less, the patient should be instructed on diet and physical activity and have an annual fasting lipid profile.
- If the LDL is greater than 100 mg/dL, appropriate clinical evaluation should be carried out and cholesterol-lowering therapy should be initiated.

Dietary Treatment

If the LDL cholesterol is above the recommended guidelines, then the first step is always dietary therapy.

- Instruct on Step I AHA diet and remeasure total cholesterol in four to six weeks and at three months. The recommendation is for the total cholesterol to be less than 200 mg/dL. If the total cholesterol goal is met, then the LDL cholesterol should be checked to confirm reaching the LDL goal. If the LDL goal is met, then the cholesterol should be remeasured four times in the first year and twice a year there-after. Dietary and behavior modifications should be reinforced.
- If the cholesterol goal is not met, then the patient should be referred to a registered dietician for counseling and retrial on Step I diet. If cholesterol goal is still not met, then Step II diet should be used. A minimum of six months of diet is used to obtain cholesterol goals. Cholesterol levels should be checked every six to twelve weeks while trying to obtain the goals. If cholesterol goal is met, LDL level should be determined to see if LDL goal is met. If LDL goal is met, do long-term monitoring as noted at the end of the previous paragraph.
- If the cholesterol goal is not achieved, consider drug therapy. See Tables 13.1 and 13.2.

Drug Therapy

- Maximal efforts at dietary therapy should be made before initiating drug therapy and should be continued even if drug therapy is needed.

Table 13.1 Profile of Currently Used Lipid-Lowering Agents

Drugs	Total Cholesterol	LDL Cholesterol	HDL Cholesterol	Triglycerides
Gemfibrozil Capsules, USP (Lopid®)	↓	↓	↑ ↑	↓ ↓
Lovastatin (Mevacor®)	↓ ↓	↓ ↓	↔	↓
Cholestyramine Resin Powder (Questran®)	↓ ↓	↓ ↓	↔	↑
Colestipol HCI Granules (Colestid®)	↓ ↓	↓ ↓	↔	↑
Probucol Tablets (Lorelco®)	↓ ↓	↓ ↓	↓	↔
Clofibrate (Atromid-S®)	↓ or ↔	↑ or ↓	↑ or ↔	↓ ↓
Niacin Tablets (nicotinic acid) (Nicolar®)	↓	↓	↑ or ↓	↓ ↓

LDL, low-density lipoprotein; HDL, high-density lipoprotein
↑, increase; ↑↑, greater increase; ↓, decrease; ↓↓, greater decrease; ↔, no effect

Table 13.2 Effect of Medication on Specific Blood Lipids

Drug	Primary Effects on Plasma Lipids and Lipoproteins	Principal Adverse Reactions and Drug Interactions
Gemfibrozil Capsules, USP (Lopid®)	Triglycerides ↓↓ Cholesterol ↓ VLDL ↓↓ LDL ↓ HDL ↑↑	Abdominal and epigastric pain, diarrhea, nausea, vomiting. Known interaction with anticoagulants.
Cholestyramine Resin Powder (Questran®)	Triglycerides ↑ Cholesterol ↓↓ VLDL ↑ LDL ↓↓ HDL ↔	Constipation, nausea, bloating. Decreased absorption of fat-soluble vitamins (A, D, and K) and other drugs, delaying or reducing their absorption.
Colestipol HCl Granules (Colestid®)	Triglycerides ↑ Cholesterol ↓↓ VLDL ↑ LDL ↓↓ HDL ↔	Constipation, nausea, bloating. Decreased absorption of fat-soluble vitamins (A, D, and K) and other drugs, delaying or reducing their absorption.
Probucol Tablets (Lorelco®)	Triglycerides ↔ Cholesterol ↓↓ VLDL ↔ LDL ↓↓ HDL ↓	Diarrhea, abdominal pain, nausea, headache, rash. Prolongation of QT interval, decreases HDL cholesterol.
Clofibrate (Atromid-S®)	Triglycerides ↓↓ Cholesterol ↓ or ↔ VLDL ↓↓ LDL ↑ or ↓ HDL ↑ or ↔	Nausea, diarrhea, GI upset, flu-like symptoms, myalgia. Known interactions with anticoagulants.
Niacin Tablets (nicotinic acid) (Nicolar®)	Triglycerides ↓↓ Cholesterol ↓ VLDL ↓↓ LDL ↓ HDL ↑ or ↓	Severe, generalized flushing, pruitus/dry skin, GI disorders, hyperuricemia. Abnormal liver function tests.
Lovastatin (Mevacor®)	Triglycerides ↓ Cholesterol ↓↓ VLDL ↓ LDL ↓↓ HDL ↔	Nausea, gas, diarrhea, constipation, abdominal pain, dyspepsia, rash, headache. Lens opacities—slit lamp tests recommended at start of treatment and once a year thereafter. Liver function tests recommended every 4–6 weeks for at least 15 months of treatment.

HDL, high-density lipoprotein; LDL, low-density lipoprotein; VLDL, very-low-density lipoprotein; ↑, increase; ↑↑, greater increase; ↓, decrease; ↓↓, greater decrease; ↔, no effect

- The panel set the LDL levels at which drug treatment is started in such a way as to create a protective barrier to the inappropriate overuse of cholesterol-lowering drugs.
- Patients with LDL cholesterol of 190 mg/dL or greater, and those with LDL cholesterol 160–189 mg/dL who also have two CHD risk factors, should be considered for drug therapy.
- The bile acid sequestrants and nicotinic acid are considered the drugs of first choice. Both Questran and nicotinic acid have been shown to lower CHD risk in clinical trials, and their long-term safety has been established.
- HMG CoA reductase Inhibitors are in a new class of drugs. These drugs are very effective in lowering LDL cholesterol, but their long-term safety has yet to be established.
- The other available drugs—Lorelco, Lopid, and Colestid—are not as effective in lowering LDL cholesterol as are the drugs of first choice or lovastatin. The goals of drug therapy are the same as those of dietary therapy.
- Drug therapy is likely to continue for a lifetime.
- Cholesterol is an active area of research. Ongoing and future investigations can be expected to expand and refine drug treatment options.
- If cholesterol goal is not achieved with diet and a first-line drug, then a different drug or combination should be used. If cholesterol goal is still not reached, a lipid specialist should be consulted.
- If LDL goal is achieved on drug therapy, then total cholesterol should be monitored every four months and LDL measured annually.

- Each person is different, so both dietary and drug treatment should be individualized. Overall coronary heart disease risk status should be carefully monitored and changed where appropriate.

MOST SIGNIFICANT MODIFICATIONS OF THE ORIGINAL 1987 GUIDELINES

In those persons with known atherosclerotic cardiovascular disease (coronary artery disease, carotid artery disease, peripheral vascular disease), LDL cholesterol levels of less than 100 should be the desired goal. This generally correlates to a total cholesterol level of 170 or less.

All persons over the age of twenty should have at least one lipid profile where total cholesterol, HDL cholesterol, and LDL cholesterol levels are determined.

14

Eating Away from Home

Eating away from home is a common part of the American lifestyle. This may be due to established routines, necessity, convenience, or pleasure. Whatever the reason, you can certainly continue eating out and maintain the healthy low-fat diet you've worked to establish. In many ways, eating a low-fat meal away from home has become easier in recent years. With the increased awareness of cholesterol and saturated fats, many patrons of restaurants have been requesting low-fat food selections. Today, you will find meals that follow the American Heart Association guidelines in many restaurants and on some airlines. These approved items or meals have some special designation on the menu. When you see these items, usually designated by an "AHA approved" or a heart on the menu, it will be easy for you to select a low-fat meal away from home. But what if the restaurant of your choice doesn't have these menu keys? Don't despair. With a little thought and planning, you can make selections that follow the guidelines you have learned in this book.

Here are a few suggestions to remember when you go to a restaurant for a low-fat meal. Remember, everything you have learned to this point still applies. You may want to phone the restaurant before going, to inquire if they have low-fat, low-cholesterol menu items or if they are willing to substitute on request. Once you arrive, take your time to examine the menu. Choose items that are low in saturated fats. As a patron of the restaurant, you are the customer, and the customer is *always* right. Don't be intimidated by the menu, the surroundings, or the personnel. Ask how food is prepared and request any necessary changes. If you have made a particular request and the food is not prepared or served accordingly, you should send it back. Be assertive, not aggressive, in your requests.

This chapter will provide you with guidelines on how to eat away from home while continuing to adhere to a good low-saturated-fat diet. If the restaurant does not have healthy-heart food choices, request that they consider adding these types of meals to their menus.

WHAT TO LOOK FOR ON THE MENU

Certain words or phrases are used to describe food preparation that will help you spot low-fat selections. The following lists are quick references. The first two lists include descriptions and methods of preparing food that should be low in saturated fat. The last two lists describe methods of food preparation which are most likely to be poor low-fat food choices. The remainder of this chapter will give you more detailed information on restaurant eating. Included will be information on all types of dining, from fast-food to elegant restaurants and ethnic eateries.

CHOOSE THESE METHODS OF FOOD PREPARATION
Baked
Broiled
Poached
Roasted
Steamed

SELECT THESE DESCRIPTIONS OF PREPARATION
In wine
In tomato juice
Dry-broiled (in lemon juice or wine)
Fresh from the garden

AVOID SELECTIONS WITH THE FOLLOWING DESCRIPTIONS
Fried, pan-fried, or in its own gravy
Braised
Buttered, buttery, or in butter sauce
Creamy, creamed, in cream sauce, or hollandaise
Crispy
Cheese sauce, escalloped, au gratin, parmesan, or cheesy
Basted, sautéed, or marinated in oil or butter

TYPES OF DISHES TO AVOID
Casseroles
Hash
Meat or potpies
Stews

HOW TO BEGIN TO CHOOSE

Sometimes, with all the many choices presented on a menu, it is easy to be overwhelmed and confused. Don't panic or worry. The same rules for a good low-saturated-fat diet that you have been learning all along still apply. If you will be selecting several courses, it is probably wise to make your entree choice first. Even though you may be having an appetizer, salad, or soup first, don't make that your first selection from the menu. You will find it easier to select the entree and build the rest of the meal around it. That means that you will want to choose an entree that is preferably turkey, chicken, fish, or nonmeat. You will find it best to limit your perusal of the menu to just those items. Looking at menu items that you have no intention of selecting tends to make the decision process more difficult than it needs to be. Examine the entree items that fit the low-fat category and determine how they are prepared. Continue to think about saturated fats just as you do when grocery shopping. The part of the menu that describes the preparation is like looking at the ingredient list on a label (and you're now a pro at label reading!). If the menu does not describe the preparation process, ask your server. Remember, you are the customer! If the item is prepared in a way that makes it an unwise low-fat choice, you may be able to request a change in preparation. Low-fat eating is becoming more of a norm in the United States, and since restaurants are frequently asked to alter the preparation of menu items, don't be bashful. You are not the first and won't be the last patron to make that request. An example of preparation substitution might be a breast of chicken that is broiled with wine and butter. Certainly, the breast of chicken is a low-saturated-fat choice, and broiled with wine would be an excellent selection. The butter in addition to the wine adds unnecessary saturated fats to this item. Ask the server if the same selection could be prepared without the butter, using just wine or replacing the butter with margarine. If those changes in preparation can be accommodated, then the item would be a wise choice. If you select an entree that is simple in its preparation, it is probably a better low-fat choice. Choose items that are broiled or baked and have a simple but tasty basting. Healthful, low-fat meals can be tasty and delicious so don't settle for anything less. Pick your entree first and remember to limit menu-gazing to just the selections that are good low-fat choices. Now that the entree has been chosen, go back and select the rest of the meal.

Choosing the Rest of the Meal

After the entree has been selected, it is easier for most people to choose the rest of the meal. Salads are excellent low-fat, low-calorie additions, or sometimes a meal in themselves. Greens, vegetables, and fruits make delicious low-fat salads. Stay away from eggs, meats, and toppings like bacon and croutons. The popularity of salad bars has made it possible for you to be selective in the creation of your salad, and many offer a wide variety of choices. If a salad bar is not available, you may request that eggs, meat, bacon, or croutons be eliminated in the preparation, or simply remove the unwanted items from your salad when it arrives. When ordering a salad, request that the dressing be served on the side. You will then be able to control the amount that is added. Often a perfectly good and healthful salad is drowned in a high-calorie, high-fat dressing. Try lemon juice, oil and vinegar, or a fat-free dressing. When using a rich dressing, add a little lemon juice, vinegar, or water to dilute it and use sparingly. Salads can be an excellent low-fat, low-cholesterol accompaniment to any meal. Enjoy!

Do Appetizers Fit into a Healthful, Low-Fat Meal?

Absolutely! You can enjoy fresh fruits and melons or raw vegetables as appetizers. Additionally, steamed or raw seafood is an excellent choice for starting a meal. There is no need to deprive yourself of an appetizer because you are on a low-fat food plan. Just pick the ones that are appropriate. A word of caution to those of you who must watch your calorie intake to achieve or maintain your ideal weight: You may want to think twice about using calories for an appetizer and "save" them for the main event, or even dessert. The choice is yours, so decide which will give you the most satisfaction. If you do decide to start your meal with an appetizer, you may satisfy your need with vegetables without spending too much of your calorie allowance.

Appetizers can make an evening of dining out an even more special event. There are many low-fat choices that you can enjoy and continue to eat for a healthy heart. You will want to stay away from crackers, spreads, and chips. As you have seen in some of the label reading, these items tend to contain hydrogenated fats and often palm and/or coconut oil. Choose your appetizers wisely for both fat and calorie content, and get ready to have a wonderful time. Enjoy your meal!

Soup as Part of a Low-Fat Die

There are many wonderful s
but you must be careful. You can p
soup at home by substituting ingredie
the preparation, but soup selections can
when eating out. (See the recipes containe
ter 16 for additional information.) There a
problems that you should consider when orde
soup in a restaurant. First of all, you can not make
quests for the soup to be prepared in a specific way, a
you often can with other parts of the meal. Since soups
are made in large quantity and are served in portions
from the pot, this means that you will not be able to
have your soup prepared with skim milk instead of
whole milk or heavy cream, for example. Therefore,
soups listed as "creamed," "cream of," or "creamy"
should be avoided when making your selection. Soups
frequently contain ingredients that are prepared with
fats and/or egg yolks. For example, soups containing
noodles, dumplings, or matzo balls probably contain
fats and eggs and should not be selected when dining
out. Soup selection in a restaurant can be done; it just
requires a little discrimination and thought. If you
have any questions about the preparation of the soup,
ask your server. The information you receive will help
you make a better choice.

Once again, limit your consideration of the menu
to only the soups that would be wise low-fat, low-cholesterol choices. You can select from either hot or cold
soups. Hot soup on a cold day can be something that is
especially good and satisfying. And cold soups can really hit the spot in the heat of the summer. Choose a
soup that is clear or is listed as a broth or a consommé
on the menu. These are usually good low-fat soups

cold fruit and ices as long as hen dining out on, but you can l of soup with

oups you can enjoy, prepare almost any nts and altering be a bit tricky d in Chap- e some ring a re-

r" in reference hanging. Nei- t are thinking tter has both

cholesterol and saturated fat and should be avoided. But what about bread? When eating out, limit your intake of breads. Most breads do contain eggs, milk, and butter. Once again, you will have many more options when baking at home. For example, you can replace whole eggs with egg whites or egg substitutes, skim milk can be used instead of whole milk, and margarine can be used in place of butter in your recipes. (See recipes in Chapter 16 for further information.) When eating at a restaurant, you do not have to give up the bread or breadsticks, but use your judgment and limit how much you eat. If you do eat the bread, avoid using butter. Ask for margarine and use it sparingly. Both the bread and margarine contain calories that you may prefer eating in the entree, dessert, or beverage. The choice is yours to make, so "spend" your calories in the way that will give you the most pleasure. Bread, breadsticks, and margarine can all be enjoyed when dining at home or out, but eat them in moderation.

Rolls, pastry, and Danish all belong to the "bread" family on the menu but in reality ought to be thought of in the "fat" family. These items usually contain more butter and sometimes additional egg yolks. Also, some rolls, pastry, and Danish contain cheese. Obviously, all of these items should be avoided or at least limited.

Would You Care for a Dessert?

Sure, why not! You can have a wonderful low-cholesterol, low-fat dessert without feeling deprived. With your increased awareness of cholesterol, you will find that dessert items on the menu have changed in recent years. How many times have you ended a perfectly delicious meal by overindulging in a high-fat dessert? Do you remember how you felt after eating that dessert? All too often, desserts with lots of whipped cream, chocolate, or sauces make you uncomfortable. When that happens, you find that you didn't really enjoy the dessert after all. You can eliminate that too-full feeling by choosing a low-fat, low-cholesterol dessert to top off your meal to perfection. You don't have to eliminate dessert as there are plenty of good low-fat choices available. One way you can enjoy dessert is by finishing your meal with fresh fruit. Please don't add whipped cream or toppings, either dairy or nondairy. Many of the dairy toppings are made from whole milk and cream. The nondairy toppings frequently contain palm or coconut oils. Fresh fruit finishes your meal with a nice sweet taste without adding fats or a lot of calories. Choosing an out-of-season fruit or an exotic variety may be just the special touch that your dining-out experience should have.

You don't want fruit for dessert? There are other good low-fat choices for you. Maybe a cool refreshing ice or sherbet will suit your taste. Or how about an angel food cake with or without fruit topping? These are all good low-cholesterol, low-fat desserts you can enjoy. Remember that your selection for desserts prepared at home are increased a hundredfold by making appropriate substitutions in the preparation of the recipe. But when eating out you can still find a good dessert selection with a little discrimination. Go ahead, order dessert, and sit back and relax after that wonderful healthy-heart meal you've just enjoyed.

What about Drinks?

Many times drinks are not mentioned when discussing cholesterol. However, there are some cholesterol considerations. The first consideration is that alcoholic beverages add calories. Although alcohol does not contain cholesterol or saturated fat, it does contain calories. You know that one important way to lower and control cholesterol is by maintaining ideal body weight. You may certainly choose to have an alcoholic beverage, but you must adjust your meal to accommodate the additional calories. You may want to minimize the calories by diluting the alcohol; that way you can enjoy more for less. One way to do just that is by drinking a wine spritzer instead of a glass of wine. When the wine is diluted with a low-calorie seltzer or soda, you can reduce the calorie content to almost half and still have all of the enjoyment. If you do not want to use your calories on alcohol but want to have something fun and delicious, you may try a low-calorie sparkling water with a lime, lemon, or orange slice.

In addition to the calorie aspect of the alcoholic beverage, you must remember that alcohol raises triglyceride levels. If you have elevated triglycerides, you should avoid alcohol or at least dilute it as we have suggested above. You can dilute wine and "hard liquor," but most people do not dilute beer. Light beers still raise the triglyceride level in your blood. Only the calories are reduced. It is the reduction of calories that allows the beer to be labeled as light. You will have to read the label to determine the calorie content, as each product is a bit different. The fact that alcohol raises triglycerides must be considered when discussing a low-cholesterol, low-fat diet.

The final consideration when ordering an alcoholic beverage is to avoid the popular ice-cream drinks and specialty liquors. While the piña colada may taste good, it is not good for your heart. Not only is it made with ice cream, but it also contains coconut, both of which are high in saturated fat. Remember that ice cream contains saturated fat, whether it is in a bowl or in a drink. To follow a healthful low-fat diet plan, you should avoid ice-cream drinks because they are sources of saturated fat. Specialty liquors such as Irish cream may in fact contain cream or milk products. You should check the labels of your favorite liquors and find substitutions if they contain these cholesterol-raising ingredients. A no-fat spritzer or soda can be the perfect accompaniment to any meal at home or while you are dining out.

Fast-Food Restaurants

It is confusing, and in some cases almost impossible, to try to figure out how much fat is in a fast-food item and how it is prepared. We have included an extensive listing of fast-food restaurants in the appendix. Restaurants are listed with their menu items and the fat content for each item. You will find it helpful and easy to look up any particular item for a fast-food chain by referring to the tables in Appendix 3. But here are some general tips to remember about fast-food eating and the selections you will make.

If you are going to be eating out at a fast-food restaurant, there's no need to complain that the menu contains no items low in fat and cholesterol. Most of the national fast-food restaurant chains have selections that can fit into a low-cholesterol, low-fat diet. Changing times have given you alternatives to the "greasy" fast foods we used to associate with these places. Most fast-food establishments now have salads offered on their menus, either prepared or as salad bars. Take advantage of the salad bars to create your own low-fat salad or meal. Remember to stay away from the eggs, meats, bacon, and croutons. At a salad bar you can add the exact amount of dressing you want. Once again, oil and vinegar or lemon juice are the best low-fat dressings. Some restaurants offer low-fat and/or low-calorie dressings, and these may be good choices for you. Even when the salad is prepared and served to you, the dressing is usually contained in a packet and served on the side. Many of these packets list the ingredients so you can analyze the contents for yourself.

Salads aren't the only new item on fast-food menus. You can now get vegetables and baked potatoes instead of the old standard french fries. If you do choose the baked potato, top it with margarine or yogurt in place of the butter and sour cream. Some fast-food restaurants also offer baked potatoes topped with vegetables. The vegetables are great as long as they don't come with cheese sauce.

Many chicken products have been added to the fast-food menu. But not all of these additions are as healthful as the advertisers would have you think. Chicken products served at fast-food eateries are sometimes fried in beef fat and lard (check the tables in Appendix 3). If that is the case, stay away from the chicken at these places. Chicken fried in vegetable oil is better than that fried in beef fat or lard, but not by much. The chicken is still fried, and you know that is not a good low-fat method of preparation. Baked breast of chicken sandwiches are found at some fast-food restaurants, and these would be the best choice if available.

When eating at fast-food restaurants, stay away from the hamburgers, especially those that are fried. Cheeseburgers are a poor choice because they add more saturated fat in the cheese, in addition to the beef, which may be fried. You can request skim milk at most fast-food places if you want a milk product. Some milk shakes and malts are actually good choices, as they are made from ice milk or non-fat yogurt.

Fast-food eating is improving. It is much easier to eat a low-fat meal today at a fast-food restaurant than it was even two or three years ago. As the general public becomes more aware of cholesterol, you will probably see additional changes in the menus at fast-food places. Speak up and let the big companies know you want to be able to get a fast, low-fat meal at their restaurants. Changes have been made because of public demand, and certainly still more will be made. Remember, you are the customer!

Italian Food

If you think pasta when you say Italian, you are thinking low-fat, low-cholesterol foods. Pastas can be good items for the cholesterol-conscious eater as long as the pasta is not filled with cheeses or meats. Stay away from pasta and Italian dishes that have cream sauces or butter. The sauces that are listed as marinara (made with tomatoes, onions, and garlic) and marsala (made with wine) are both tasty and low in fat. Linguini with clam sauce, either red or white, is an Italian low-fat speciality, as is pasta primavera. If pasta is not appealing to you, many Italian dishes are prepared with chicken or fish. Choose an item that is simply prepared and, again, avoid selections that use cheeses and creams.

Chinese Food

Many selections on the menu at Chinese restaurants make good low-fat choices. Dishes that are steamed or lightly stir-fried in vegetable oil can be excellent healthy-heart meals. This is particularly true if it is a vegetable, chicken, or seafood selection. Ask that sauces and soy be served on the side. That way you can add just a small amount or none at all, depending on your taste.

The menu at most Chinese restaurants offers you a variety of low-fat, low-cholesterol choices, but it is not without pitfalls. There are items you should avoid or limit when eating Chinese food. Avoid the Egg Foo Yung and all items served in Lobster Sauce. Both of these selections are made with egg yolks. Main dishes that are deep-fried should also be avoided. However, it is more likely that items in a Chinese restaurant will be stir-fried rather than deep-fried. Steamed rice is a better selection than fried rice, which generally contains eggs and may be fried in butter. Ask the server if you have any questions about the preparation. Noodles should be limited. Some soups should be limited due to the addition of these noodles, while others should be avoided due to the eggs used in the preparation.

The meat served in Hunan and Szechuan-style Chinese cooking is first fried in hot oil and then prepared. For this reason it is best to eliminate these types of foods when adhering to a low-fat food plan. As you have learned, chicken and fish or seafood dishes are generally better low-fat choices than beef or pork.

Japanese Fare

Japanese food, for the most part, is low in cholesterol and saturated fats. The dishes that are listed as "yakimono" are good choices for your low-cholesterol diet as those items have been broiled. The sashimi (raw fish) and sushi (raw fish and rice) are both superb low-cholesterol, low-fat choices. Many traditional Japanese dishes feature vegetables and/or tofu, which is a soybean curd protein that does not contain cholesterol. By and large, Japanese foods, with the exception of tempura, which is prepared by deep-frying, are good when following a low-cholesterol diet.

Mexican Food

There are choices for the person interested in limiting cholesterol and saturated fat when eating Mexican. Some items on the menu will fit into a low-fat diet, but not the tortilla chips and refried beans. These are both fried in lard and therefore contain large amounts of saturated fat and cholesterol. With these exceptions, there is a whole menu of low-fat vegetable, bean (not refried), chicken, and fish dishes from which to choose. Burritos are made with flour tortillas that are not made with lard and are not fried and would be a good choice. Ask that sour cream, dressings, guacamole, and cheese be served on the side so that you can control their use or eliminate them completely if you choose. So if Mexican suits your taste, there is plenty to choose from without adding fat to your diet.

French Cuisine

Yes, you can eat at French restaurants and still adhere to your low-cholesterol, low-fat diet. Probably the most important guideline to remember when eating French cuisine is "make it simply delicious." This means good food with simple preparation. Many French dishes are wonderful blends of herbs and spices used in baking or broiling chicken and fish. These would be good low-fat selections. Look for food with simple preparations and the creative use of herbs when making selections at a French restaurant. Menu items that have been broiled with wine are often very tasty, low-fat selections. French cooking is frequently synonymous with sauces and creams. This is just the thing you will want to avoid. The sauces that are used in French cuisine are made with egg yolks, milk, and butter. For example, hollandaise is made with egg yolks and butter, bechamel with milk and butter, bearnaise with egg yolks, and mousseline with egg yolks, butter, and heavy cream. Dishes that are listed as "nouvelle cuisine" or "nouvelle sauces " may have reduced calorie content and are generally lighter because flour has been eliminated or reduced in the preparation, but they contain saturated fats and cholesterol. For this reason the nouvelle selections should be critically examined to determine if they would be wise heart-smart choices.

If a dish is prepared in an acceptable way and the sauce is added after cooking, you may be able to have the sauce held and the dish served without garnish. If you have any questions about the preparation of a dish you are considering, ask your server how it is prepared. Stay away from menu items that are described as au gratin. They will be served with cheese and butter topping.

For dessert you are probably wisest to stay with a fresh fruit selection or a refreshing sorbet. Do not be tempted by the heavy creams and pastries that are usually displayed in French restaurants. Remember, they will only lead to blocking your arteries.

French eating is possible on a low-cholesterol, low-fat diet, but it will take some planning and thought on your part. Enjoy your meal, be good to your heart, and keep it simply delicious!

15

Miscellaneous Subjects

This chapter contains limited information on multiple subjects that many people may have heard of and have questions about. It is not intended to be an indepth discussion, but should be helpful.

Antioxidants. Scientific studies suggest that cholesterol is oxidized (changed by a chemical reaction) prior to it being able to enter the arterial wall. There is evidence to suggest that stopping the chemical reaction, that is, oxidation, will prevent plaque formation (atherosclerosis) from occurring. There are several naturally occurring antioxidants, including vitamins A, E, C, and beta carotene. In addition, several drugs have been shown to have antioxidant properties. Although a large number of people take these vitamins on a daily basis, their benefit has not yet been proven in clinical studies. In addition, the long-term effect of large doses of vitamins is still unknown. The role of antioxidants in preventing atherosclerosis is promising.

Chelation therapy. EDTA (edetate disodium) chelation therapy for atherosclerosis is very controversial. This process involves the intravenous infusion of agents that tend to bind and remove calcium, zinc, lead, iron, and copper. Treatments are usually given several times per week for a total of 20 to 40 treatments. Theoretically, the infusions remove calcium from the atherosclerotic plaques. At the same time, the removal of iron and copper stops the enzymes which cause oxidation of cholesterol. Unfortunately, there is no hard scientific evidence that chelation therapy is beneficial. Most reports in the scientific literature are testimonials, not large double-blinded studies. At this time, only one well-designed clinical trial is in the literature. In this study, 153 patients with severe claudication (pain in the legs because of decreased blood flow secondary to arterial blockages) were placed in a placebo group or a group that received EDTA for twenty treatments over 5 to 9 weeks. No statistical difference was found in the two groups as far as their maximum walking distance without pain or pain-free periods. Presently, the American Heart Association does not believe that chelation therapy has been shown to be beneficial. Most physicians do not recommend this treatment. Adverse effects, including kidney failure, bone marrow depression, and heart rhythm irregularities, have occurred with EDTA treatment. These side effects apparently are rare when infusions are given at recommended rates and doses.

Circadian rhythm. There is an internal clock that controls the body's functions over a 24-hour period. Not much is known about this other than it exists in humans and all animals. If you are used to waking up at the same time every morning, you still wake up at the same time in the morning even if you don't set the alarm clock. This is your internal clock. It is hard to reset your internal clock. That why "jet lag" occurs when you travel a long distance (change many time zones) in a short time. Cholesterol levels do show some variation related to circadian rhythm or time of day. These tend to be rather minor. Larger but still minor variations in cholesterol level are seen by season.

Diurnal variation. Diurnal variation just relates to the day-night cycle variations in living things. It is essentially the same as circadian rhythm, which is explained above.

Garlic. Interestingly, garlic has been shown to favorably alter blood cholesterol levels in humans and decrease induced atherosclerosis in animals. How garlic lowers cholesterol levels is unknown. There is much interest in garlic, and more information may be available in the near future. It appears eating garlic or taking garlic tablets may be helpful in lowering blood cholesterol levels, and no information suggests any risk or danger associated with garlic. The following verse may sum things up fairly well.

Garlic

"Sith Garlicke then hath power to save from death,
Bear with it though it make unsavoury breathe,
And scorne not Garlicke like some that thinke
It only makes men winke and drinke and stinke."
—Sir John Harington (1607)

Gene Therapy. The greatest promise for treatment advances of hyperlipidemia and many other diseases is gene therapy. Gene therapy is only useful in those people who have a genetic defect which causes a disease or disorder to occur. In people with hyperlipidemia, there can be many different genetic disorders that cause a necessary enzyme to be absent or present in less than normal amounts. Enzymes are helper substances necessary for a chemical reaction or conversion to occur. Gene therapy can also help correct a problem where receptors on cells are decreased or absent. Cell receptors are proteins which allow certain substances (such as cholesterol) to enter cells for internal (cellular) use or conversion. Many times, these genetic disorders are the most serious problems and are the hardest to treat adequately. You must remember that most problems of hyperlipidemia in the U.S. are caused by dietary problems, not genetic disorders. However, for those people with genetic disorders of lipid metabolism, gene therapy holds great promise.

Homocysteine. All proteins are made of building blocks called amino acids. Essential amino acids are those amino acids that must be consumed as they can not be made by the metabolism of other substances or amino acids. Homocysteine is an amino acid found in the body. It is not an essential amino acid, as it is an intermediate metabolic product from the essential amino acid methionine. There is much evidence that blood homocysteine levels correlate to atherosclerosis levels. This would suggest that homocysteine may be a causative factor in atherosclerosis. It is believed that homocysteine is actually toxic (a poison) to the lining cells of blood vessels (endothelium). The possibility of a relationship between homocysteine and atherosclerosis was first proposed in 1908. Since then, many scientific studies have suggested that this may be true. Because of recent advances in ways to measure homocysteine blood levels, scientific studies should be easier to perform. The good news is that homocysteine blood levels can usually be decreased to normal levels by several vitamins. These include folate, pyridoxine, and vitamin B_{12}. Much research remains to be done, but homocysteine appears to be a significant factor in the development of atherosclerosis. If this is proven to be true, then treating the homocysteine blood level may have a significant effect on reducing the occurrence or severity of atherosclerosis.

Plasmapheresis. It is possible to physically remove the LDL cholesterol from blood by running it through a special type of filter that binds the LDL cholesterol. This requires being connected to a machine that circulates the patient's blood into the filter and then back to the patient. This process is termed plasmapheresis and is given in a simplified description here. Plasmapheresis is performed in people with very high LDL cholesterol levels that can not be reasonably controlled with medications and diet. Usually, plasmapheresis can only be done at specialized lipid centers. Using this method, LDL cholesterol can be lowered 40–80%, but plasmapheresis must be done on a regular basis to maintain this reduction.

Regression. Several scientific studies now suggest that it may be possible to cause atherosclerotic plaques or blockages to become less severe. It is believed that these plaques show regression because cholesterol and triglycerides are removed from the plaques and transported back into the bloodstream. Regression has been shown to occur when the LDL cholesterol is below 100 mg/dL. This usually corresponds to a total cholesterol of 170 or less. Controlling cholesterol to these levels almost certainly helps prevent progression or worsening of blockages in the arteries.

Trans fatty acids. When liquid vegetable oils have hydrogen added to them to make them solids, they are called hydrogenated or partially hydrogenated. The more "hydrogenated" the liquid oils are, the harder or more solid they become. These partially or totally hydrogenated oils are called trans fatty acids. They behave like saturated fats in that they cause the blood cholesterol level to rise. The more hydrogenated an oil is, the more like a saturated fat it becomes. Therefore, softer margarines (less hydrogenated) are better for you than harder margarines, which are more hydrogenated.

16 Cooking Tips to Lower Saturated Fat and Cholesterol

Now that you know the difference in the types of fats and the recommended limitations in your diet, let's put this knowledge to practical use in your own kitchen. Once again, a major consideration is that you must first be a smart shopper. If you do not have the proper low-fat ingredients in your home, you will not make the necessary changes to get control of your cholesterol. With the right ingredients and a few changes in your recipes, it will be easy to serve delicious, heart-smart meals.

We will start with our modifications with meats. Meats are sources of saturated fats. Your primary focus in converting recipes to low-fat is reducing and limiting the saturated fat. In selecting meats, remember that fish, chicken, and turkey most often have lower saturated-fat content. You can frequently substitute chicken or turkey in dishes calling for beef or pork. For instance, if the recipe calls for hamburger, you can use ground turkey with the same results and less saturated fat (see recipes included in this chapter). You should limit your use of beef, pork, lamb, or veal to no more than three times a week. When you do use beef, pork, or lamb, start with a lean cut, that is with little marbling and without visible fat. Even lean cuts of meat contain saturated fat. Extra care must be taken so that the meat will be prepared in a manner that will minimize the addition of saturated fat to a nice lean choice. Use a rack to broil, roast, or bake. This allows the fat to drain, and therefore less is absorbed back into the meat. Use a low temperature for a longer period of time when roasting or baking. This is referred to as slow-roasting. Slow-roasting will allow more fat to cook out and drain away from the meat. Cooking at high temperatures tends to seal the meat so the fat is retained. While slow-roasting will help facilitate the removal of the fat from the meat, this will also tend to dry the meat. Therefore it is very important to frequently baste, to keep the meat moist while cooking at low temperatures. Baste with wine, fruit juices, non-oil-based marinades, fat-free or low-fat meat broths. Do not baste with the drippings, as this contains the saturated fats. When breading a meat prior to roasting, use a no- or low-fat breading and only lightly coat the meat. Breading adds calories and, if heavily applied, will seal the meat and thus promote the retention of saturated fats. Do not fry meats. Frying adds saturated fat and additionally allows the meat to absorb its own fat, which could be removed by choosing a different cooking method. If a recipe calls for a meat to be browned, you can bake it, then carefully place it under the broiler to achieve the browning. When you use low-fat cooking by both the selection of lean cuts and the method of preparation, it is imperative to remember that fat adds both flavor and moisture to foods.

With that in mind, you must pay special attention to the fact that you will have to add moisture to your low-fat recipes (as we discussed with frequent basting) as well as flavor. The addition of flavor can be accomplished with the use of herbs and seasonings. If you keep your low-fat foods moist and flavorful, you will never miss the fat.

Chicken and turkey are excellent low-fat meat substitutes. However, certain processing procedures can change these low-fat meats into highly saturated fat foods. An example of this is self-basting turkey. These turkeys are prepared by injecting fat and/or butter under the skin. This has two major problems. The first is that the skin is left on the turkey (to make turkey a good low-fat choice, the skin must be removed before cooking). The second problem is that the turkey self-bastes in the additional fat that has been injected as well as its own natural fat. You can buy a fresh turkey, remove the skin, and the bake it in wine, fruit juice, or no-fat chicken broth and have a delicious dish that minimizes the saturated fat. Another example of a perfectly good low-fat choice that becomes a saturated fat nightmare are prepared meals with breaded turkey or chicken. Many of the breaded foods will remove the skin, which is a good step, but then they coat the chicken or turkey in a breading that contains palm or coconut oil along with other hydrogenated or partially hydrogenated oils. This breading then takes a good low-fat choice and adds unnecessary fats and calories. We have also just discussed that breading tends to hold fats in the meat instead of allowing them to drain away during the cooking process. (All of this information on breading pertains to fish products as well.)

You can prepare delicious soups, stews, and gravies with reduced saturated fat by removing the fat from the meat juices to prepare low-fat stock. This can be done by cooking the meat a day ahead of time. Refrigerate the meat juice overnight. The saturated fat will harden on the top. Skim the hardened fat from the juice and you have a good low-fat broth. If you do not have time to prepare the meat a day ahead of time, you can simply add an ice cube to harden the fat and skim it from the top. Additionally, fat removers are available commercially. They look like a measuring cup with the spout to pour located low in the cup. This method also works to skim fat from the meat juice. Once the fat has been removed by any of these methods, simply prepare the dish as directed. Once again, remember that when fat is removed, flavor is reduced. Since you will want to make your stocks and gravies as flavorful as possible, this will mean using herbs, seasonings, or flavors.

MEATS AND FISH

Foods to Use	Turkey and chicken (skinless)
	Fish
	Canned fish packed in water
Use in Moderation	Lean cuts beef, pork, lamb, and veal
	Shellfish (shrimp, lobster, etc.)
Foods to Avoid	Marbled beef
	Processed pork products (bacon, sausage, etc.)
	Processed meats (hot dogs, luncheon meats)
	Fatty fowl (duck, goose)
	Organ meats (liver, kidneys, brains, etc.)
	Fish canned in oil
	Self-basting turkeys
	Breaded fish and poultry products

Ice cream is a dairy product that most of us love and certainly enjoy from time to time. Ice cream has a high butterfat content. In some products, the butterfat is as much as 45–50%. Just look at that bowl of ice cream and think that it is half fat! But don't despair. There are many low-fat and no-fat substitutes available. Some examples of good low-fat substitutes are ice milks and frozen yogurt. Be sure that you read the label before you bring these products into your home. Some ice milks and frozen yogurts contain palm and coconut oil. Obviously these would not make good low-fat choices. There are also new substitutes called frozen dessert products. Many of these are no-fat substitutes for ice cream. Read the labels and experiment to find a product that will satisfy your taste needs. It seems as though every day new low-fat or no-fat substitutes make their way to our grocery shelves. You will have to test various product to see if they meet your taste standards. Not everyone's tastes are the same. If they were, there would not be as many choices available. Take a chance and look for new ways to satisfy your taste. What may be good to me might be a terrible choice for you.

USE	AVOID
Skim milk	Whole milk
Low-fat cheeses	Whole milk cheeses
No-fat or low-fat yogurt	Creamy high-fat yogurt
Evaporated skim milk	Evaporated milk
Liquid nondairy creamer	Heavy cream
Low-fat yogurt Non-fat sour cream	Sour cream
Egg substitutes Egg whites	Whole eggs

USE	AVOID
Ice milk	Ice cream
Frozen no-fat yogurt	
No-fat frozen dessert	
Low-fat sweetened condensed milk	Sweetened condensed milk

COOKING WITH FATS AND OILS

The majority of saturated fat that you ingest comes from three categories of foods: meat and meat products, dairy foods, and fats. We have just examined meat and dairy products and their appropriate low-saturated-fat substitutions. Now we will tackle the fat category. To determine which fats are highly saturated, you will want to keep in mind the two rules that you learned in Chapter 4. If it comes from an animal source or is solid at room temperature, it contains saturated fat. Again, we stress that the exceptions are palm and coconut oils. Both are high in saturated fat even though they are from a vegetable source and can be liquid. With that in mind, look at your eating habits and examine your recipes for ways to decrease your saturated fat intake and control the unsaturated fats. Your best substitutions will be made by choosing vegetable products that contain no palm or coconut oil and are liquid.

What kind of fats do you use that are highly saturated? Any fat that comes from an animal source is certainly a saturated fat. That includes butter, lard, bacon drippings, chicken fat, cream sauces, and drippings from all meat preparation. Secondly, any fat product that is solid at room ternperature contains saturated fat. Some examples of that would be shortening and margarine. You can substitute any of these with a good low-saturated-fat choice. Using a liquid vegetable oil would be an excellent low-saturated-fat choice since it is both liquid and vegetable in origin. Canola oil has the lowest amount of saturated and the highest mono-unsaturated fat available (including the omega 3 type) so would be the best choice as a substitute (see Chapter 4). Another alternative is safflower oil. Safflower oil is very low in saturated fats, but instead of high amounts of monounsaturated fats, it contains high levels of polyunsaturated fats (see Chapter 4). Some people find the taste of safflower oil bitter and do not choose to use it. Give safflower oil a try because it is the highest polyunsaturated and low in saturated fat. If it is not to your liking, many other vegetable oils are available. You may have to test several different products to find the one that suits your own particular taste.

You will find that sometimes a liquid is inappropriate as a substitute for the saturated fat. For example, you wouldn't want to put oil on toast. In these cases you will want to use a low saturated fat in a solid form, like margarine. Margarine is made from a vegetable, usually corn, but it is solid at room temperature. It meets one of the two criteria for a good low-saturated fat, but not both. This means that margarine has less saturated fat than butter, but more than vegetable oil. Once you decide to use a margarine, you must then decide if it should be stick or soft. Since margarine is from vegetable fat, the only other consideration is the solidity factor. Stick margarine is harder so contains more trans fatty acids. Your best margarine choice, therefore, is soft margarine. It's a little like the old saying: "Good, better, best. Don't let it rest till your good is better and your better is your best." Oil is the best fat choice you can make, as long as it is not palm or coconut oil. Soft margarine is the better choice, and stick is a good choice. Whenever you can, use oil for your cooking or in recipes. If oil is not appropriate, then soft margarine would be the next best choice. If you cannot use soft margarine, then stick would be better than butter or some other animal saturated fat. It will take some experimenting to find which oil and soft margarine taste better to you. But isn't it nice to have so many low-saturated choices available? You will find some recipes in this chapter that have been adapted and use low-saturated-fat substitutes. To make it easy for you to do this with your own family's favorite recipes, use the conversion guide on page 155.

The final source of saturated fat we would like to discuss is chocolate or any form of cocoa butter. Both cocoa butter and the chocolate that is made from it contain saturated fat. Cocoa powder and carob contain saturated fat, but in very reduced amounts in comparison to chocolate. Look for chocolate products that are made from either cocoa powder or carob. Chocolate can be replaced in many of your recipes by substituting cocoa powder and polyunsaturated oil. One ounce of baking chocolate contains 8.4 grams of saturated fat. By comparison, three tablespoons of cocoa powder combined with one tablespoon of vegetable oil contains .8 grams of saturated fat and produces the same results.

You have learned how to make good, low-fat substitutions in your buying and eating habits. Making changes in your eating patterns is not something you can do overnight. The saying—every little bit helps—can be applied to your efforts to reduce saturated fat from your diet. Whenever you choose a low-saturated-fat product, you are helping to reduce the amount of fat in your coronary arteries. The war against heart disease is fought with each food choice you make. Every little step helps, and pretty soon you have a lot of little steps toward making big strides in keeping your heart healthy. Be patient with yourself in making these substitutions and changes. Above all, keep trying!

Use the following substitutions of oils for fats:

USE	IN PLACE OF
⅞ cup of polyunsaturated oil or 1 cup soft or tub margarine or 1 cup (2 sticks) margarine	1 cup butter
3 tablespoons cocoa powder plus 1 tablespoon polyunsaturated oil	1 ounce baking chocolate
polyunsaturated oil or soft margarine or stick margarine	shortening, lard, bacon fat, chicken fat, or meat drippings

DELICIOUS LOW-FAT RECIPES

These recipes are included in this book to give you examples of how to begin thinking about altering your current recipes to make them good low-fat selections. Many low-cholesterol recipe books are currently on the market to help you add to the meals you are now preparing. We think it is a more beneficial approach to learn to adapt the recipes you use and like. For that reason we have selected some recipes that represent different types of dishes that you may already be serving. However, these recipes are prepared in a low-cholesterol, low-saturated-fat way.

Soups

EGG DROP SOUP

Traditionally, Egg Drop Soup is made with whole eggs and occasionally additional egg yolks. Our Egg Drop Soup uses egg substitute and still delivers all of the rich full taste of the traditional soup, but without cholesterol.

4 cups water	$\frac{1}{4}$ teaspoon tarragon
4 cubes low sodium chicken bouillon	$\frac{1}{4}$ cup egg substitute
3 tablespoons cornstarch	

Bring $3\frac{1}{2}$ cups water to boil in a medium saucepan. Add chicken bouillon to boiling water. Stir until bouillon is dissolved. Combine the cornstarch with the remaining $\frac{1}{2}$ cup water. Add the cornstarch mixture to the dissolved bouillon, stirring constantly. Mix in tarragon. Cook over medium heat until thickened and boiling. Continue to cook for one minute longer. Reduce heat to low and slowly add egg substitute in a thin stream. Do not stir while adding the egg substitute. Cook for about one minute. Stir once before removing from heat. Serves 6.

HALIBUT BISQUE

Bisques are usually made with heavy creams, milk, and butter, which are high-cholesterol and saturated-fat foods. You can enjoy all of the flavor of a bisque without the fat and cholesterol-containing ingredients by using substitutes. Try our version of Halibut

Bisque, a delicious, creamy creation. You can also substitute shrimp or lobster for the halibut.

2 tablespoons chopped onion	dash salt
2 tablespoons chopped celery	¼ teaspoon paprika
¼ cup soft margarine, melted	dash pepper
2 tablespoons flour	1 quart liquid nondairy creamer
	¾ pound cooked flaked halibut
	¼ teaspoon nutmeg

Cook onion and celery in margarine in a pot until tender and onions are clear. Blend in flour and all seasonings except nutmeg. Stir in nondiary creamer gradually. Cook until thickened, stirring constantly. Add halibut. Cook over low heat for 30–45 minutes, stirring occasionally. Garnish with nutmeg. Serves 6.

CHICKEN STOCK

There are many recipes for preparing chicken stock. This one is rich in flavor and low in fats and salt. This easy chicken stock can be prepared in quantity and then frozen for uses in different ways. You will find many ways of using the chicken stock in recipes. One example follows.

5 pounds skinless chicken	⅓ cup diced carrots
3 quarts water	⅓ cup diced onion
2 sprigs parsley	½ cup diced celery
¼ teaspoon thyme	dash salt
1 crumbled bay leaf	fresh ground pepper

In a pot, combine chicken and water. Bring to a slow boil. Skim any fat off top of water. Add all remaining ingredients. Cover and simmer over low heat. Cook approximately 3½ hours. Skim fat from top prior to cooling. Yield: 2½ quarts.

Many low-fat ingredients may be added to the basic chicken stock to create some wonderful low-fat soups. Here's an example:

MATZO BALL SOUP

These low-fat, low-cholesterol matzo balls are light and fluffy without the eggs and chicken fat generally associated with them. Add these matzo balls to your chicken stock for a delicious hot soup.

¼	cup cold water	1	egg white
2	tablespoons soft margarine	½	cup matzo meal
		¼	teaspoon salt
¼	cup egg substitute	6	cups chicken stock

Combine water, margarine, egg substitute, and egg white in a bowl. Add matzo meal, stirring constantly. Blend in salt. Cover and refrigerate for 30 minutes. Warm chicken stock over medium heat. Take cooled matzo mixture from refrigerator and drop rounded teaspoonfuls on top of just boiling chicken stock. Cover and cook at a slow boil for 20 minutes. Serve piping hot. Serves 4.

Chicken and Turkey Dishes

Thousands of recipes contain chicken and turkey. The recipes that follow in this section are to give you an idea of the tremendous variety of dishes that can be prepared using chicken and turkey, some of which you may only associate with beef or pork. Once again the important consideration in this section is for you to adapt your recipes and make them good low-cholesterol, low-fat meals.

CRISPY SOUTHERN CHICKEN

Usually southern chicken is coated with the skin on and fried in shortening. This recipe gives you that crispy coating and juicy taste you love without the fat and cholesterol.

3 pounds skinless chicken	1 cup cornflake crumbs
salt, pepper to taste	
1 cup skim milk	canola oil cooking & baking spray

Preheat oven to 400° F. Season chicken to taste. Dip chicken in milk and shake off excess. Thoroughly coat chicken with the cornflake crumbs. Let chicken sit to allow coating to adhere to chicken before placing in baking dish. Spray the baking dish with oil. Place chicken in dish. Bake for 45 minutes. Chicken will be tender, juicy, and crispy. Serves 4.

CHICKEN KABOBS

6 chicken breasts, skinless and deboned
12 small cherry tomatoes
2 medium onions, quartered
12 mushrooms

Cut chicken breasts into pieces for the skewers. Alternate chicken, tomatoes, onions, and mushrooms on skewer. Place skewers in marinade (recipe follows) for about 30 minutes.

CHICKEN KABOB MARINADE

½ cup canola oil   ⅛ teaspoon pepper
1 clove garlic, crushed   ⅛ teaspoon lemon juice
1 tablespoon vinegar

Mix all ingredients together. Place marinade in a glass baking dish. Do not use a metal pan. Place chicken kabobs in marinade. After kabobs have marinated for 30 minutes, cook either under broiler or on grill. Cook 10 to 15 minutes, turning and basting with marinade at least twice during cooking. Serves 6.

GROUND TURKEY CHILI

Once you try this hearty turkey chili, you will be convinced that low-fat meals can be better than the old high-saturated-fat variety.

Canola oil cooking & baking spray
¼ cup chopped onion
1 clove garlic, minced
1 pound ground turkey
2 cans (15 ounces *each*) tomato sauce
2 cans (15 ounces *each*) kidney beans
1 can (6 ounces) tomato paste
3 tablespoons chili powder
¼ teaspoon oregano
¼ teaspoon paprika
chopped onions and tomatoes (garnish)

Spray a medium skillet with oil, then sauté onion and garlic until tender and soft over medium heat. Add ground turkey to onion and garlic mixture. Cook ground turkey slowly and break up frequently. If you are not used to cooking with ground turkey, it becomes a white-gray color as it cooks. It does not brown as ground beef does. In a large pot combine tomato sauce, kidney beans, tomato paste, chili powder, oregano, and paprika. Add ground turkey mixture to tomato sauce and cook, covered, over low heat for 1½ to 2 hours, stirring occasionally. Serve topped with chopped onions and tomatoes. Serves 8.

Ground turkey can be used in most recipes that call for ground beef. Try it in your meatballs or meat sauce and spaghetti. Turkey meatloaf is a hearty delicious meal. Use the same recipes that you have for years. Just substitute good low-fat meats, oils, and margarines for the beef, pork, lard, shortening, and butter. You will find that most of your favorite dishes are completely adaptable and are lighter and full of flavor.

TURKEY MARSALA

This is an elegant meal that will impress your friends and relatives at any dinner party. It is easy to prepare and quite inexpensive, but the results are magnificent.

2 pounds turkey cutlet	½ cup marsala
½ cup flour	3 tablespoons beef consommé
canola oil cooking & baking spray	½ pound mushrooms, sliced
1 tablespoon soft margarine	1 tablespoon flour (optional)

Pound turkey cutlets between two pieces of waxed paper until ¼ inch thick. Do not dry cutlet prior to flouring. Dredge cutlet through flour. Shake off excess flour. Spray the skillet with oil and heat until water skittles across the skillet. Add cutlet to hot skillet; turn once when edges become white. Continue to cook until cutlet becomes lightly browned. Do not overcook cutlets as they will become tough. Cutlets cook very quickly, so watch carefully. When cutlets are browned, remove from skillet. Add margarine, marsala, consommé, and mushrooms to the skillet and cook over medium heat. If the sauce is too thin, you may flour to thicken. Add flour slowly, stirring constantly. When sauce is smooth, add cutlets; stir and coat until covered. Serve immediately. Serves 8.

CREAMY YOGURT CHICKEN

1 cup fine bread crumbs

1/4 cup grated Parmesan cheese

1 tablespoon dried onion

1 teaspoon garlic powder

1/4 teaspoon oregano

1/4 teaspoon thyme

1/4 teaspoon fresh ground pepper

1/2 teaspoon seasoned salt

4 skinned chicken breasts

8 ounces plain no-fat yogurt

1/4 cup melted margarine

2 teaspoons sesame seeds

Creamy Yogurt Sauce (recipe follows)

On a plate, mix together the first eight ingredients on the left (down to and including seasoned salt). Rinse chicken, coat with yogurt. Roll yogurt-coated chicken in bread crumb and seasoning mixture. Place chicken breast meaty side up in baking pan. Drizzle melted margarine on top of chicken. Sprinkle with sesame seeds and bake, uncovered, at 375° for 50 minutes.

CREAMY YOGURT SAUCE

8 ounces plain no-fat yogurt

1 can (10.75 ounces) Campbell's Healthy Request Cream of Chicken Soup

1 teaspoon lemon juice

½ teaspoon Worchestershire sauce

½ teaspoon garlic powder

½ teaspoon seasoned salt

¼ cup no-fat chicken broth

Place all ingredients in saucepan and cook over medium heat. Stir frequently until hot. Pour sauce over chicken to serve. Serves 4.

Desserts

The following are some examples of good heart-smart desserts you can make at home. These recipes are easy and delicious. You don't have to deprive yourself of dessert just because you are on a low-fat food plan. There are many low-fat cookbooks on the market if you are interested in adding to your recipes. Remember, you may be able to make substitutions and changes in the recipes you currently use.

LOW-FAT WHIPPED CREAM SUBSTITUTE

1 teaspoon Knox gelatin

3 tablespoons boiling water

¾ cup nonfat dry milk (which contains no palm or coconut oil)

½ cup ice water

4 tablespoons sugar

3 tablespoons Canola oil

Place gelatin in boiling water and dissolve completely, stirring continuously. Allow the gelatin mixture to cool to room temperature. While gelatin mixture is cooling, put a deep narrow mixing bowl into the freezer for approximately 15 minutes. Mix milk and ice water in the bowl from freezer and blend together at high speed. Using high speed, slowly add sugar to milk mixture. When the mixture takes on a creamy appearance, begin to add the gelatin mixture. After completely blending the gelatin mixture, at high speed, slowly drizzle the oil into the mixture. Freeze overnight and then place in refrigerator for at least four hours prior to serving.

STRAWBERRY CREAM PIE

This cool and refreshing low-fat dessert will delight your family and impress your friends.

1 pint fresh strawberries
1 package (4-serving size) instant vanilla pudding
1 cup no-fat sour cream
¼ cup skim milk
2 teaspoons grated orange or lemon peel
3½ cups low-fat whipped cream substitute (page 163)
   graham cracker pie crust

Hull berries and set aside. Combine instant pudding, sour cream, milk, and citrus peel. When combined, add 2 cups topping. Beat with wire wisk until well blended, about one minute. Spoon half of filling into pie crust. Arrange berries on filling and press down. Add remaining half of filling. Freeze for one hour or chill for three hours before serving. Garnish with additional strawberries and whipped topping. Makes one 9-inch pie.

ALL-PURPOSE PIE CRUST

2 cups flour
1 teaspoon salt
¼ cup canola oil
¼ cup + 1 tablespoon cold water

In a large mixing bowl, sift flour and salt. Mix oil and water together until foamy and add to flour and salt mixture. Blend well. Divide into two equal portions. Roll out crust on waxed paper. Place one rolled-out dough into 10-inch pie pan. After adding pie filling, use the second portion of the dough for the top crust or another pie. Yield: two 10-inch pie crusts.

FUDGY BROWNIES

canola oil cooking spray
¼ cup oil
½ cup egg substitute
¾ cup sugar
1 teaspoon vanilla extract
½ cup all-purpose flour
6 tablespoons unsweetened carob powder or Nestle Quik
½ teaspoon baking powder
½ cup chopped walnuts (optional)

Preheat oven to 350° F. Spray bottom and sides of 8-inch square baking dish with canola oil spray. Combine oil, egg substitute, sugar, and vanilla in a large mixing bowl. Do not sift flour. Blend in flour, carob, and baking powder. Stir in nuts if desired. Pour batter into prepared baking dish. Bake 15 to 20 minutes or until a toothpick inserted into center comes out clean. Cool completely before cutting into squares. Makes 16 brownies.

POUND CAKE

1   package (8 ounces) no-fat cream cheese
½   cup margarine
1   cup sugar
1½   teaspoons vanilla
8   ounces egg substitute
2   cups flour
1½   teaspoons baking powder
     canola oil baking spray

Preheat oven to 325° F. Combine cream cheese, margarine, and sugar. Mix well until smooth. Add vanilla and egg substitute slowly while mixing on low speed. Slowly add flour and baking powder. Continue to use the low speed of an electric mixer until fully blended. Pour into loaf pan that has been sprayed with oil. Bake for 1 hour and 15 minutes to 1 hour and 20 minutes. Cool and remove from pan. Serves 16.

Snacks

PITA TRIANGLES

pita bread
no-fat Italian salad dressing
grated part-skim Parmesan cheese

Cut pita bread into triangles. Pour no-fat Italian dressing into a bowl. Dip pita triangles into salad dressing and arrange on a cookie sheet. Sprinkle Parmesean cheese lightly on top of triangles. Place in a 350° F oven to lightly crisp pita and lightly brown cheese.

VEGGIE DIP

1   cup plain no-fat yogurt
3   green onions, chopped
$\frac{1}{4}$ teaspoon dill weed
$\frac{1}{8}$ teaspoon garlic powder

Combine all ingredients with mixer or blender. Refrigerate and serve with veggies and pretzels.

Appendix 1

Flow Charts for the Treatment of Adults Based on Cholesterol Blood Tests

Figure 1 **Dietary Recommendations for High Blood Cholesterol**

Nutrient	Recommended Intake
Total fat	30% or less of total calories
Saturated fat	8–10% of total calories
Polyunsaturated fat	Up to 10% of total calories
Monounsaturated fat	Up to 15% of total calories
Cholesterol	Less than 300 mg/day
Total calories	To achieve and maintain desirable weight

Figure 2   Primary Prevention in Adults Without Evidence of CHD: Initial Classification Based on Total Cholesterol and HDL Cholesterol

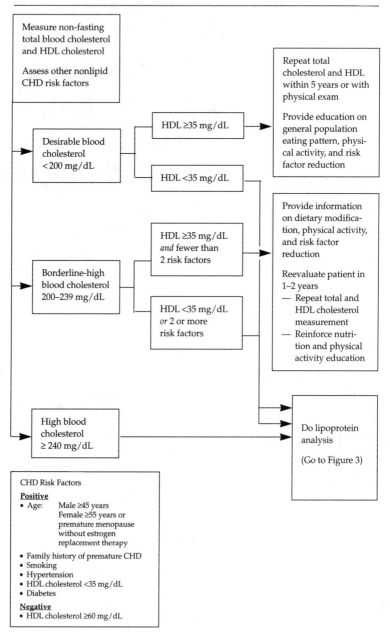

Figure 3 Primary Prevention in Adults Without Evidence of CHD: Subsequent Classification Based on LDL Cholesterol

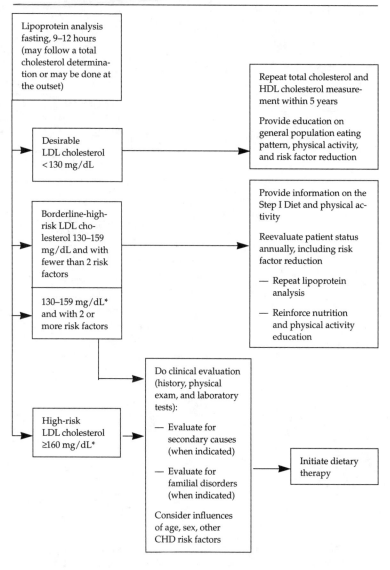

*On the basis of the average of two determinations. If the first two LDL cholesterol tests differ by more than 30 mg/dL, a third test should be obtained within 1–8 weeks and the average value of three tests used.

Figure 4 Secondary Prevention in Adults With Evidence of CHD: Classification Based on LDL Cholesterol

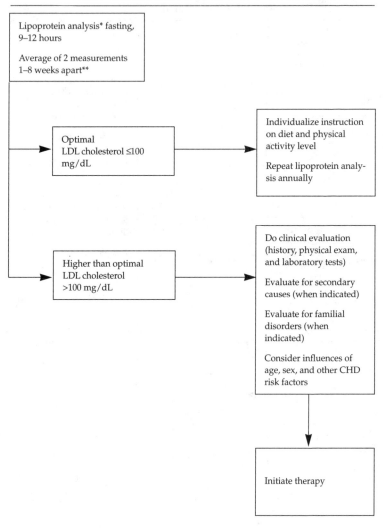

*Lipoprotein analysis should be performed when the patient is not in the recovery phase from an acute coronary or other medical event that would lower their usual LDL cholesterol level.

**If the first two LDL cholesterol tests differ by more than 30 mg/dL, a third test should be obtained within 1–8 weeks and the average value of the three tests used.

Appendix 2

Saturated Fat, Cholesterol, Total Fat, and Calorie Content of Foods

When controlling cholesterol, it is essential to know the saturated fat and cholesterol content of foods. The following charts list the saturated fat, cholesterol, total fat, percent of calories from fat and total calories for many foods. These tables are arranged into particular types of food to make it easier to find a certain item.

MEATS

Meats are a major source of saturated fat and cholesterol in the diet. The following list includes various cuts of beef, lamb, pork, and veal. Use lean cuts of meat and prepare utilizing the suggestions in Chapter 16 to reduce the saturated fat content.

Product (3½ Ounces, Cooked)*	Saturated Fatty Acids (Grams)	Cholesterol (Milligrams)	Fat[1] (Grams)	Calories From Fat[2] (%)	Total Calories
Beef					
Kidneys, Simmered[3]	1.1	387	3.4	21	144
Liver, Braised[3]	1.9	389	4.9	27	161
Round, top round, lean only, broiled	2.2	84	6.2	29	191
Round, eye of round, lean only, broasted	2.5	69	6.5	32	183
Round, tip round, lean only, roasted	2.8	81	7.5	36	190
Round, full cut, lean only, choice, broiled	2.9	82	8.0	37	194
Round, bottom round, lean only, braised	3.4	96	9.7	39	222
Short loin, top loin, lean only, broiled	3.6	76	8.9	40	203
Wedge-bone sirloin, lean only, broiled	3.6	89	8.7	38	208
Short loin, tenderloin, lean only broiled	3.6	84	9.3	41	204
Chuck, arm pot roast, lean only, braised	3.8	101	10.0	39	231
Short loin, T-bone steak, lean only, choice, broiled	4.2	80	10.4	44	214

*3½ ozs = 100 grams (approximately)

[1]Total fat = saturated fatty acids plus monounsaturated fatty acids plus polyunsaturated fatty acids.

[2]Percent calories from fat = (total fat calories divided by total calories) multiplied by 100; total fat calories = total fat (grams) multiplied by 9.

[3]Liver and most organ meals are low in fat, but high in cholesterol. If you are eating to lower your blood cholesterol, you should consider your total cholesterol intake before selecting an organ meat.

Product (3½ Ounces, Cooked)*	Saturated Fatty Acids (Grams)	Cholesterol (Milligrams)	Fat[1] (Grams)	Calories From Fat[2] (%)	Total Calories
Short loin, porter-house steak, lean only, choice, broiled	4.3	80	10.8	45	218
Brisket, whole, lean only, braised	4.6	93	12.8	48	241
Rib eye, small end (ribs 10-12), lean only, choice, broiled	4.9	80	11.6	47	225
Rib, whoel (ribs 6-12), lean only, roasted	5.8	81	13.8	52	240
Flank, lean only, choice, braised	5.9	71	13.8	51	244
Rib, large ends (ribs 6-9), lean only, broiled	6.1	82	14.2	55	233
Chuck, blade roast, lean only, braised	6.2	106	15.3	51	270
Corned beef, cured, brisket, cooked	6.3	98	19.0	68	251
Flank, lean and fat, choice, braised	6.6	72	15.5	54	257
Ground, lean, broiled medium	7.2	87	18.5	61	272
Round, full cut, lean and fat, choice, braised	7.3	84	18.2	60	274
Rib, short ribs, lean and fat, choice, braised	7.7	93	18.1	55	295
Salami, cured, cooked, smoked, 3-4 slices	9.0	65	20.7	71	262
Short loin, T-bone steak, lean and fat, choice, broiled	10.2	84	24.6	68	324
Chuck, arm pot roast, lean and fat, braised	10.7	99	26.0	67	350

Product (3½ Ounces, Cooked)*	Saturated Fatty Acids (Grams)	Cholesterol (Milligrams)	Fat[1] (Grams)	Calories From Fat[2] (%)	Total Calories
Sausage, cured, cooked, smoked, about 2	11.4	67	26.9	78	312
Bologna, cured, 3-4 slices	12.1	58	28.5	82	312
Frankfurter, cured, about 2	12.0	61	28.5	82	315
Lamb					
Leg, lean only, roasted	3.0	89	8.2	39	191
Loin chop, lean only, broiled	4.1	94	9.4	39	215
Rib, lean only, roasted	5.7	88	12.3	48	232
Arm chop, lean only, braised	6.0	122	14.6	47	279
Rib, lean and fat, roasted	14.2	90	30.6	75	368
Pork					
Cured, ham steak, boneless, extra lean, unheated	1.4	45	4.2	31	122
Liver, braised[3]	1.4	355	4.4	24	165
Kidneys, braised[3]	1.5	480	4.7	28	151
Fresh, loin, tenderloin, lean only, roasted	2.4	48	7.0	37	170
Cured, shoulder, arm picnic, lean only, roasted	2.4	48	7.0	37	170
Cured, ham, boneless, regular, roasted	3.1	59	9.0	46	178
Fresh, leg (ham), shank half, lean only, roasted	3.6	92	10.5	44	215
Fresh, leg (ham), rump half, lean only, roasted	3.7	96	10.7	43	221

Product (3½ Ounces, Cooked)*	Saturated Fatty Acids (Grams)	Cholesterol (Milligrams)	Fat[1] (Grams)	Calories From Fat[2] (%)	Total Calories
Fresh loin, center loin, sirloin, lean only, roasted	4.5	90	13.2	50	236
Fresh, loin, center rib, lean only, roasted	4.8	79	13.8	51	245
Fresh, loin, top loin, lean only, roasted	4.8	79	13.8	51	245
Fresh, shoulder, blade, Boston, lean only, roasted	5.8	98	16.8	59	256
Fresh, loin, blade, lean only, roasted	6.6	89	19.3	62	279
Fresh, loin, sirloin, lean and fat, roasted	7.4	91	20.4	63	291
Cured, shoulder, arm picnic, lean and fat, roasted	7.7	58	21.4	69	280
Fresh, loin, center loin, lean and fat, roasted	7.9	91	21.8	64	305
Cured, shoulder, blade roll, lean and fat, roasted	8.4	67	23.5	74	287
Fresh, Italian sausage, cooked	9.0	78	25.7	72	323
Fresh, bratwurst, cooked	9.3	60	25.9	77	301
Fresh, chitterlings, cooked	10.1	143	28.8	86	303
Cured, liver sausage, liverwurst	10.6	158	28.5	79	326
Cured, smoked link sausage, grilled	11.3	68	31.8	74	389
Fresh, spareribs, lean and fat, braised	11.8	121	30.3	69	397
Cured, salami, dry or hard	11.9	—	33.7	75	407

— = information not available in the sources used.

Product (3½ Ounces, Cooked)*	Saturated Fatty Acids (Grams)	Cholesterol (Milligrams)	Fat[1] (Grams)	Calories From Fat[2] (%)	Total Calories
Bacon, fried	17.4	85	49.2	78	576
Veal					
Rump, lean only, roasted	—	128	2.2	13	156
Sirloin, lean only, roasted	—	128	3.2	19	153
Arm steak, lean only, cooked	—	90	5.3	24	200
Loin chop, lean only, cooked	—	90	6.7	29	207
Blade, lean only, cooked	—	90	7.8	33	211
Cutlet, medium fat, braised or broiled	4.8	128	11.0	37	271
Foreshank, medium fat, stewed	—	90	10.4	43	216
Plate, medium fat, stewed	—	90	21.2	63	303
Rib, medium fat, roasted	7.1	128	16.9	70	218
Flank, medium fat, stewed	—	90	32.3	75	390

Sources:

Composition of Foods: Beef Products - Raw • Processed • Prepared, Agricultural Handbook 8-13. United States Department of Agriculture, Human Nutrition Information Service (August 1986).

Composition of Foods: Pork Products - Raw• Processed • Prepared, Agricultural Handbook 8-10. United States Department of Agriculture, Human Nutrition Information Service (August 1983).

Home and Garden Bulletin. Nutritive Value of Foods. No. 72. United States Department of Agriculture. Human Nutrition Information Service (1986).

POULTRY

Poultry is generally lower in saturated fat and cholesterol than most cuts of meat. This is especially true when the skin has been removed. The following table gives saturated fat, cholesterol and calorie content of several selections of chicken and turkey.

Product (3½ Ounces, Cooked)*	Saturated Fatty Acids (Grams)	Cholesterol (Milligrams)	Fat[1] (Grams)	Calories From Fat[2] (%)	Total Calories
Turkey, fryer-roasters, light meat without skin, roasted	0.4	86	1.9	8	140
Chicken, roasters, light meat without skin, roasted	1.1	75	4.1	24	153
Turkey, fryer-roasters, light meat with skin, roasted	1.3	95	4.6	25	164
Chicken, broilers or fryers, light meat without skin, roasted	1.3	85	4.5	24	173
Turkey, fryer-roasters, dark meat without skin, roasted	1.4	112	4.3	24	162
Chicken, stewing, light meat without skin, stewed	2.0	70	8.0	34	213
Turkey roll, light and dark	2.0	55	7.0	42	149

*3½ ozs = 100 grams (approximately)
[1]Total fat = saturated fatty acids plus monounsaturated fatty acids plus polyunsaturated fatty acids.
[2]Percent calories from fat = (total fat calories divided by total calories) multiplied by 100; total fat calories = total fat (grams) multiplied by 9.

Product (3½ Ounces, Cooked)*	Saturated Fatty Acids (Grams)	Cholesterol (Milligrams)	Fat[1] (Grams)	Calories From Fat[2] (%)	Total Calories
Turkey, fryer-roasters, dark meat with skin, roasted	2.1	117	7.1	35	182
Chicken, roasters, dark meat without skin, roasted	2.4	75	8.8	44	178
Chicken, broilers or fryers, dark meat without skin, roasted	2.7	93	9.7	43	205
Chicken, broilers or fryers, light meat with skin, roasted	3.0	84	10.9	44	222
Chicken, stewing, dark meat without skin, stewed	4.1	95	15.3	53	258
Duck, domesticated, flesh only, roasted	4.2	89	11.2	50	201
Chicken, broilers or fryers, dark meat with skin, roasted	4.4	91	15.8	56	253
Goose, domesticated, flesh only, roasted	4.6	96	12.7	48	238
Turkey bologna, about 3½ slices	5.1	99	15.2	69	199
Chicken frankfurter, about 2	5.9	107	17.7	70	226

Source:

Composition of Foods: Poultry Products - Raw • Processed • Prepared, Agricultural Handbook 8-5. United States Department of Agriculture, Science and Education Administration (August 1979).

FISH AND SHELLFISH

To help lower cholesterol, you will want to include more fish and shellfish in your diet. Fish and shellfish are lower in saturated fat than meat or poultry. Some shellfish, however, do contain cholesterol and their use should be limited to meet the cholesterol limitations. Omega-3 fatty acids are found in fish and shellfish and have been shown to be beneficial in reducing cholesterol. (See Chapter 4.) This table gives the saturated fat, cholesterol, Omega-3 fatty acids, total fat, calories from fat, and total calorie content of selected fish and shellfish.

Product (3½ Ounces, Cooked)*	Saturated Fatty Acids (Grams)	Cholesterol (Milligrams)	Omega-3 Fatty Acids (Grams)	Fat[1] (Grams)	Calories From Fat[2] (%)	Total Calories
Finfish						
Haddock, dry heat	0.2	74	0.2	0.9	7	112
Cod, Atlantic, dry heat	0.2	55	0.2	0.9	7	105
Pollock, walleye, dry heat	0.2	96	1.5	1.1	9	113
Perch, mixed species, dry heat	0.2	42	0.3	1.2	9	117
Grouper, mixed species, dry heat	0.3	47	—	1.3	10	118
Whiting, mixed species, dry heat	0.3	84	0.9	1.7	13	115
Snapper, mixed species, dry heat	0.4	47	—	1.7	12	128
Halibut, Atlantic and Pacific, dry heat	0.4	41	0.6	2.9	19	140
Rockfish, Pacific, dry heat	0.5	44	0.5	2.0	15	121
Sea bass, mixed species, dry heat	0.7	53	—	2.5	19	124

*3½ ozs. = 100 grams (approximately).

[1]Total fat = saturated fatty acids plus monounsaturated fatty acids plus polyunsaturated fatty acids.

[2]Percent calories from fat = (total fat calories divided by total calories) multiplied by 100; total fat calories = total fat (grams) multiplied by 9.

— = Information not available in sources used.

Product (3½ Ounces, Cooked)*	Saturated Fatty Acids (Grams)	Cholesterol (Milligrams)	Omega-3 Fatty Acids (Grams)	Fat[1] (Grams)	Calories From Fat[2] (%)	Total Calories
Trout, rainbow, dry heat	0.8	73	0.9	4.3	26	151
Swordfish, dry heat	1.4	50	1.1	5.1	30	155
Tuna, bluefin, dry heat	1.6	49	—	6.3	31	184
Salmon, sockeye, dry heat	1.9	87	1.3	11.0	46	216
Anchovy, European, canned	2.2	—	2.1	9.7	42	210
Herring, Atlantic, dry heat	2.6	77	2.1	11.5	51	203
Eel, dry heat	3.0	161	0.7	15.0	57	236
Mackerel, Atlantic, dry heat	4.2	75	1.3	17.8	61	262
Pompano, Florida, dry heat	4.5	64	—	12.1	52	211
Crustaceans						
Lobster, northern	0.1	72	0.1	0.6	6	98
Crab, blue, moist heat	0.2	100	0.5	1.8	16	102
Shrimp, mixed species, moist heat	0.3	195	0.3	1.1	10	99
Mollusks						
Whelk, moist heat	0.1	130	—	0.8	3	275
Clam, mixed species, moist heat	0.2	67	0.3	2.0	12	148
Mussel, blue, moist heat	0.9	56	0.8	4.5	23	172
Oyster, Eastern, moist heat	1.3	109	1.0	5.0	33	137

Source:
Composition of Foods: Finfish and Shellfish Products - Raw • Processed • Prepared, Agriculture Handbook 8-15. United States Department of Agriculture (in press).

DAIRY AND EGG PRODUCTS

Dairy products contain both saturated fat and cholesterol. When selecting dairy products choose those with the lowest butterfat content. Egg yolks are a major source of cholesterol. Egg whites or substitutes should be used in place of egg yolks.

Product	Saturated Fatty Acids (Grams)	Cholesterol (Milligrams)	Fat[1] (Grams)	Calories From Fat[2] (%)	Total Calories
Milk (8 ounces)					
Skim milk	0.3	4	0.4	5	86
Buttermilk	1.3	9	2.2	20	99
Low-fat milk, 1% fat	1.6	10	2.6	23	102
Low-fat milk, 2% fat	2.9	18	4.7	35	121
Whole milk, 3.3% fat	5.1	33	8.2	49	150
Yogurt (4 ounces)					
Plain yogurt, low-fat	0.1	2	0.2	3	63
Plain yogurt	2.4	14	3.7	47	70
Cheese					
Cottage cheese, low-fat, 1% fat, 4 oz.	0.7	5	1.2	13	82
Mozzarella, part-skim, 1 oz.	2.9	16	4.5	56	72
Cottage cheese, creamed, 4 oz.	3.2	17	5.1	39	117
Mozzarella, 1 oz.	3.7	22	6.1	69	80
Sour cream, 1 oz.	3.7	12	5.9	87	61
American processed cheese spread, pasteurized, 1 oz.	3.8	16	6.0	66	82

[1]Total fat = saturated fatty acids plus monounsaturated fatty acids plus polyunsaturated fatty acids.

[2]Percent calories from fat = (total fat calories divided by total calories) multiplied by 100; total fat calories = total fat (grams) multiplied by 9.

oz. = ounce

Product	Saturated Fatty Acids (Grams)	Cholesterol (Milligrams)	Fat[1] (Grams)	Calories From Fat[2] (%)	Total Calories
Feta, 1 oz.	4.2	25	6.0	72	75
Neufchatel, 1 oz.	4.2	22	6.6	81	74
Camembert, 1 oz.	4.3	20	6.9	73	85
American processed cheese food, pasteurized, 1 oz.	4.4	18	7.0	68	93
Provolone, 1 oz.	4.8	20	7.6	68	100
Limburger, 1 oz.	4.8	26	7.7	75	93
Brie, 1 oz.	4.9	28	7.9	74	95
Romano, 1 oz.	4.9	29	7.6	63	110
Gouda, 1 oz.	5.0	32	7.8	69	101
Swiss, 1 oz.	5.0	26	7.8	65	107
Edam, 1 oz.	5.0	25	7.9	70	101
Brick, 1 oz.	5.3	27	8.4	72	105
Blue, 1 oz.	5.3	21	8.2	73	100
Gruyere, 1 oz.	5.4	31	9.2	71	117
Muenster, 1 oz.	5.4	27	8.5	74	104
Parmesan, 1 oz.	5.4	22	8.5	59	129
Monterey Jack, 1 oz.	5.5	25	8.6	73	106
Roquefort, 1 oz.	5.5	26	8.7	75	105
Ricotta, part-skim, 4 oz.	5.6	25	9.0	52	156
American processed cheese, pasteurized, 1 oz.	5.6	27	8.9	75	106
Colby, 1 oz.	5.7	27	9.1	73	112
Cheddar, 1 oz.	6.0	30	9.4	74	114
Cream cheese, 1 oz.	6.2	31	9.9	90	99
Ricotta, whole milk, 4 oz.	9.4	58	14.7	67	197
Eggs					
Egg, chicken, white	0	0	tr.	0	16
Egg, chicken, whole	1.7	274	5.6	64	79
Egg, chicken, yolk	1.7	272	5.6	80	63

tr. = trace

Source:
Composition of Foods: Dairy and Egg Products - Raw • Processed • Prepared, Agriculture Handbook 8-1, United States Department of Agriculture, Agricultural Research Service (November 1976).

FATS AND OILS

Fats and oils are a major source of saturated fat in the diet. With the exceptions of lard, butter, and beef tallow, fats and oils are not sources of cholesterol. You will want to choose products with the highest polyunsaturated and lowest saturated fat content. This table lists the saturated fat, cholesterol, polyunsaturated fat, and monounsaturated fat content of selected fats and oils.

Product (1 tablespoon)	Saturated Fatty Acids (Grams)	Cholesterol (Milligrams)	Poly-unsaturated Fatty Acids (Grams)	Mono-unsaturated Fatty Acids (Grams)
Rapeseed oil (canola oil)	0.9	0	4.5	7.6
Safflower oil	1.2	0	10.1	1.6
Sunflower oil	1.4	0	5.5	6.2
Peanut butter, smooth	1.5	0	2.3	3.7
Corn oil	1.7	0	8.0	3.3
Olive oil	1.8	0	1.1	9.9
Hydrogenated sunflower oil	1.8	0	4.9	6.3
Margarine, liquid, bottled	1.8	0	5.1	3.9
Margarine, soft, tub	1.8	0	3.9	4.8
Sesame oil	1.9	0	5.7	5.4
Soybean oil	2.0	0	7.9	3.2
Margarine, stick	2.1	0	3.6	5.1
Peanut oil	2.3	0	4.3	6.2
Cottonseed oil	3.5	0	7.1	2.4
Lard	5.0	12	1.4	5.8
Beef tallow	6.4	14	0.5	5.3
Palm oil	6.7	0	1.3	5.0
Butter	7.1	31	0.4	3.3
Cocoa butter	8.1	0	0.4	4.5
Palm kernel oil	11.1	0	0.2	1.5
Coconut oil	11.8	0	0.2	0.8

BREADS, CEREALS, PASTA, RICE, DRIED PEAS, AND BEANS

The following table gives the saturated fat, cholesterol, total fat, calories from fat, and total calorie content of selected breads, cereals, pasta, rice, dried peas and beans. Select those items that are low in saturated fat and cholesterol.

Product	Saturated Fatty Acids (Grams)	Cholesterol (Milligrams)	Total Fat[1] (Grams)	Calories From Fat[2] (%)	Total Calories
Breads					
Melba toast, 1 plain	0.1	0	tr.	0	20
Pita, 1/2 large shell	0.1	0	1.0	5	165
Corn tortilla	0.1	0	1.0	14	65
Rye bread, 1 slice	0.2	0	1.0	14	65
English muffin	0.3	0	1.0	6	140
Bagel, 1, 3½" diameter	0.3	0	1.0	6	140
White bread, 1 slice	0.3	0	1.0	14	65
Rye krisp, 2 triple crackers	0.3	0	1.0	16	56
Whole wheat bread, 1 slice	0.4	0	1.0	13	70
Saltines, 4	0.5	4	1.0	18	50
Hamburger bun	0.5	tr.	2.0	16	115
Hot dog bun	0.5	tr.	2.0	16	115
Pancake, 1, 4" diameter	0.5	16	2.0	30	60
Bran muffin, 1, 2½" diameter	1.4	24	6.0	43	125

[1]Total fat = saturated fatty acids plus monounsaturated fatty acids plus polyunsaturated fatty acids.

[2]Percent calories from fat = (total fat calories divided by total calories) multiplied by 100; total fat calories = total fat (grams) multiplied by 9.

oz. = ounce

tr. = trace

Product	Saturated Fatty Acids (Grams)	Cholesterol (Milligrams)	Total Fat[1] (Grams)	Calories From Fat[2] (%)	Total Calories
Corn muffin, 1, 2$^1/_2$" diameter	1.5	23	5.0	31	145
Plain doughnut, 1, 3$^1/_4$" diameter	2.8	20	12.0	51	210
Croissant, 1, 4$^1/_2$" by 4"	3.5	13	12.0	46	235
Waffle, 1, 7" diameter	4.0	102	13.0	48	245
Cereals (1 cup)					
Corn flakes	tr.	—	0.1	0	98
Cream of wheat, cooked	tr.	—	0.5	3	134
Corn grits, cooked	tr.	—	0.5	3	146
Oatmeal, cooked	0.4	—	2.4	15	145
Granola	5.8	—	33.1	50	595
100% Natural Cereal with raisins and dates	13.7	—	20.3	37	496
Pasta (1 cup)					
Spaghetti, cooked	0.1	0	1.0	6	155
Elbow macaroni, cooked	0.1	0	1.0	6	155
Egg noodles, cooked	0.5	50	2.0	11	160
Chow mein noodles, canned	2.1	5	11.0	45	220
Rice (1 cup cooked)					
Rice, white	0.1	0	0.5	2	225
Rice, brown	0.3	0	1.0	4	230
Dried Peas and Beans (1 cup cooked)					
Split peas	0.1	0	0.8	3	231
Kidney beans	0.1	0	1.0	4	225
Lima beans	0.2	0	0.7	3	217
Black eyed peas	0.3	0	1.2	5	200
Garbanzo beans	0.4	0	4.3	14	269

— = Information not available in sources used.

Sources:

Composition of Foods: Breakfast Cereals - Raw • Processed • Prepared. Agriculture Handbook 8-16. United States Department of Agriculture, Nutrition Monitoring Division (December 1986).

Home and Garden Bulletin. Nutritive Value of Foods. No. 72. United States Department of Agriculture. Human Nutrition Information Service (1986).

SWEETS, SNACKS, AND FROZEN DESSERTS

The total dietary plan for lowering cholesterol includes limiting cholesterol, saturated fats, and weight control. To help you take control of cholesterol, the table table below lists the saturated fat, cholesterol, total fat, calories from fat, and total calorie content of common sweets, snacks, and frozen desserts.

Product	Saturated Fatty Acids (Grams)	Cholesterol (Milligrams)	Total Fat[1] (Grams)	Calories From Fat[2] (%)	Total Calories
Beverages					
Ginger ale, 12 oz.	0.0	0	0.0	0	125
Cola, regular, 12 oz.	0.0	0	0.0	0	160
Chocolate shake, 10 oz.	6.5	37	10.5	26	360
Candy (1 ounce)					
Hard candy	0.0	0	0.0	0	110
Gum drops	tr.	0	tr.	tr.	100
Fudge	2.1	1	3.0	24	115
Milk chocolate, plain	5.4	6	9.0	56	145
Cookies					
Vanilla wafers, 5 cookies, 1³/₄" diameter	0.9	12	3.3	32	94
Fig bars, 4 cookies 1⁵/₈" × 1⁵/₈" × ³/₈"	1.0	27	4.0	17	210
Chocolate brownie with icing, 1¹/₂" by 1³/₄" by ⁷/₈"	1.6	14	4.0	36	100

[1]Total fat = saturated fatty acids plus monounsaturated fatty acids plus polyunsaturated fatty acids.

[2]Percent calories from fat = (total fat calories divided by total calories) multiplied by 100; total fat calories = total fat (grams) multiplied by 9.

— = Information not available in sources used.

oz. = ounce

tr. = trace

Product	Saturated Fatty Acids (Grams)	Cholesterol (Milligrams)	Total Fat[1] (Grams)	Calories From Fat[2] (%)	Total Calories
Oatmeal cookies, 4 cookies, 2⅝" diameter	2.5	2	10.0	37	245
Chocolate chip cookies, 4 cookies, 2¼" diameter	3.9	18	11.0	54	185
Cakes and Pies					
Angel food cake, ¹/₁₂ of 10" cake	tr.	0	tr.	125	125
Gingerbread, ¹/₉ of 8" cake	1.1	1	4.0	21	175
White layer cake with white icing, ¹/₁₆ of 9" cake	2.1	3	9.0	32	260
Yellow layer cake with chocolate icing, ¹/₁₆ of 9" cake	3.0	36	8.0	31	235
Pound cake, ¹/₁₇ of loaf	3.0	64	5.0	41	110
Devils food cake with chocolate icing, ¹/₁₆ of 9" cake	3.5	37	8.0	31	235
Lemon meringue pie, ¹/₆ of 9" pie	4.3	143	14.0	36	355
Apple pie, ¹/₆ of 9" pie	4.6	0	18.0	40	405
Cream pie, ¹/₆ of 9" pie	15.0	8	23.0	46	455
Snacks					
Popcorn, air-popped, 1 cup	tr.	0	tr.	tr.	30
Pretzels, stick, 2¼", 10 pretzels	tr.	0	tr.	tr.	10
Popcorn with oil and salted, 1 cup	0.5	0	3.0	49	55
Corn chips, 1 oz.	1.4	25	9.0	52	155
Potato chips, 1 oz.	2.6	0	10.1	62	147
Pudding					
Gelatin	0.0	0	0.0	0	70

Product	Saturated Fatty Acids (Grams)	Cholesterol (Milligrams)	Total Fat[1] (Grams)	Calories From Fat[2] (%)	Total Calories
Tapioca, 1/2 cup	2.3	15	4.0	25	145
Chocolate pudding, 1/2 cup	2.4	15	4.0	24	150
Fruit popsicle, 1 bar	—	—	0.0	0	65
Fruit ice	—	—	tr.	0	247
Fudgsicle	—	—	0.2	2	91
Frozen yogurt, fruit flavored	—	—	2.0	8	216
Sherbet, orange	2.4	14	3.8	13	270
Pudding pops, 1 pop	2.5	1	2.6	25	94
Ice milk, vanilla, soft serve	2.9	13	4.6	19	223
Ice milk, vanilla, hard	3.5	18	5.6	28	184
Ice cream, vanilla, regular	8.9	59	14.3	48	269
Ice cream, french vanilla, soft serve	13.5	153	22.5	54	377
Ice cream, vanilla, rich, 16% fat	14.7	88	23.7	61	349

Sources:

Composition of Foods: Dairy and Egg Products - Raw • Processed • Prepared, Agriculture Handbook 8-1. United States Department of Agriculture, Agricultural Research Service (November 1976).

Pennington, J., and Church, H. *Bowes and Church's Food Values of Portions Commonly Used.* 14th ed. Philadelphia: J.B. Lippincott Company (1985).

Home and Garden Bulletin. Nutritive Value of Foods. United States Department of Agriculture. Human Nutrition Information Service (1986).

NUTS AND SEEDS

Choose those nuts and seeds that are lowest in saturated fats when following a low cholesterol, low-fat diet plan. This table gives you the saturated fat, cholesterol, total fat, calories from fat, and total calorie content of some nut and seed products.

Product (1 ounce)	Saturated Fatty Acids (Grams)	Cholesterol (Milligrams)	Total Fat[1] (Grams)	Calories From Fat[2] (%)	Total Calories
European chestnuts	0.2	0	1.1	9	105
Filberts or Hazelnuts	1.3	0	17.8	89	179
Almonds	1.4	0	15.0	80	167
Pecans	1.5	0	18.4	89	187
Sunflower seed kernels, roasted	1.5	0	1.4	77	165
English walnuts	1.6	0	17.6	87	182
Pistachio nuts	1.7	0	13.7	75	164
Peanuts	1.9	0	14.0	76	164
Hickory nuts	2.0	0	18.3	88	187
Pine nuts, pignolia	2.2	0	14.4	89	146
Pumpkin and squash seed kernels	2.3	0	12.0	73	148
Cashew nuts	2.8	0	13.2	73	163
Macadamia nuts	3.1	0	20.9	95	199
Brazil nuts	4.6	0	18.8	91	186
Coconut meat, unsweetened	16.3	0	18.3	88	187

[1]Total fat = saturated fatty acids plus monounsaturated fatty acids plus polyunsaturated fatty acids.

[2]Percent calories from fat = (total fat calories divided by total calories) multiplied by 100; total fat calories = total fat (grams) multiplied by 9.

Composition of Foods: Legumes and Legume Products Raw • Processed • Prepared, Agriculture Handbook 8-16. United States Department of Agriculture, Human Nutrition Information Service (December 1986).

Composition of Foods: Nut and Seed Products - Raw • Processed • Prepared, Agriculture Handbook 8-12. United States Department of Agriculture, Human Nutrition Information Service (September 1984).

MISCELLANEOUS ITEMS

The following table provides the saturated fat, cholesterol, total fat, calories from fat, and total calorie content of miscellaneous food items. This information may be beneficial to you, in adhering to a low-cholesterol, low-saturated-fat diet.

Product	Saturated Fatty Acids (Grams)	Cholesterol (Milligrams)	Total Fat[1] (Grams)	Calories From Fat[2] (%)	Total Calories
Gravies (1/2 cup)					
Au jus, canned	0.1	1	0.3	3	80
Turkey, canned	0.7	3	2.5	37	61
Beef, canned	1.4	4	2.8	41	62
Chicken, canned	1.7	3	6.8	65	95
Sauces (1/2 cup)					
Sweet and sour	tr.	0	0.1	? 1	147
Barbecue	0.3	0	2.3	22	94
White	3.2	17	6.7	50	121
Cheese	4.7	26	8.6	50	154
Sour cream	8.5	45	15.1	53	255
Hollandaise	20.9	94	34.1	87	353
Bearnaise	20.9	99	34.1	88	351
Salad Dressings (1 Tablespoon)					
Russian, low calorie	0.1	1	0.7	27	23
French, low calorie	0.1	1	0.9	37	22
Italian, low calorie	0.2	1	1.5	85	16
Thousand Island, low calorie	0.2	2	1.6	59	24
Imitation mayonnaise	0.5	4	2.9	75	35
Thousand Island, regular	0.9	—	5.6	86	59
Italian, regular	1.0	—	7.1	93	69

[1]Total fat = saturated fatty acids plus monounsaturated fatty acids plus polyunsaturated fatty acids.

[2]Percent calories from fat = (total fat calories divided by total calories) multiplied by 100; total fat calories = total fat (grams) multiplied by 9.

— = Information not available in the sources used.

Product	Saturated Fatty Acids (Grams)	Cholesterol Milligrams	Total Fat[1] (Grams)	Calories From Fat[2] (%)	Total Calories
Russian, regular	1.1	—	7.8	92	76
French, regular	1.5	—	6.4	86	67
Blue cheese	1.5	—	8.0	93	77
Mayonnaise	1.6	8	11.0	100	99
Other					
Olives, green, 4 medium	0.2	0	1.5	90	15
Nondairy creamer powdered, 1 teaspoon	0.7	0	1.0	90	10
Liquid, 1/2 oz.	less than 1 gm.	0	2.0	12.2	20
Avocado, Florida	5.3	0	27.0	72	340
Pizza, cheese, 1/8 of 15" diameter	4.1	56	9.0	28	290
Quiche lorraine, 1/8 of 8" diameter	23.2	285	48.0	72	600

Sources:

Composition of Foods: Fats and Oils - Raw • Processed • Prepared, Agriculture Handbook 8-4. United States Department of Agriculture, Science and Education Administration (June 1979).

Composition of Foods: Soups, Sauces and Gravies - Raw • Processed • Prepared, Agriculture Handbook 8-6. United States Department of Agriculture, Science and Education Administration (February 1980).

Home and Garden Bulletin. Nutritive Value of Foods. No. 72. United States Department of Agriculture. Human Nutrition Information Service (1986).

Appendix 3

Fast Food Tables

The following tables provide information about the calorie content, total fat and saturated fat content of selected fast foods. In Table One, the food items are arranged in restaurant groups. If you frequently eat at a particular fast food restaurant and would like to know about their menu items, they will be easy to find in Table One. In Table Two of the fast food information section, foods are listed according to menu items. If you are interested in eating a roast beef sandwich and want to see how various restaurants compare, you will find Table Two provides the best and easiest information.

The last portion of the fast food information section lists the addresses of several fast food chains. If you would like a complete listing of that restaurant's menu items, you can write to the address listed, or inquire at your local restaurant. Much of the calorie and fat content information for fast food restaurants, change due to different suppliers, varied cooking techniques, and substituting products. If you have any questions, ask at the local restaurant or write to the addresses listed on page 199.

Table 1

Food Product	Weight	Calories	Total Fat Grams	Saturated Fat	Fat Calories
Arby's (regular roast beef)	5 oz.	365	19	7 grams	47%
Arby's Chicken Breast Sandwich	7 oz.	567	32	7 Grams	51%
Arby's French Fries	3 oz.	222	11	3 Grams	45%
Arby's Chocolate Shake	11 oz.	426	14	7 Grams	30%
Burger King Whopper	9 oz.	584	33	13 Grams	51%
Burger King Whaler	6 oz.	478	26	3 Grams	49%
Burger King Chicken Tenders	3 oz.	223	12	3 Grams	48%
Burger King French Fries	3 oz.	255	13	5 Grams	46%
Burger King Chocolate Shake	11 oz.	351	10	5 Grams	26%
Church's Fried Chicken (2 piece)	6 oz.	487	35	9 Grams	65%
Church's Fried Chicken Fries	4 oz.	338	16	5 Grams	43%
Hardee's Roast Beef (regular)	5 oz.	338	17	6 Grams	45%
Hardee's Chicken Filet Sandwich	7 oz.	431	20	6 Grams	42%
Hardee's French Fries	3 oz.	230	12	4 Grams	47%
Hardee's Chocolate Shake	11 oz.	349	11	6 Grams	28%
McDonald's Big Mac	7 oz.	572	34	15 Grams	53%
McDonald's Filet-O-Fish	4 oz.	415	23	5 Grams	50%
McDonald's Chicken McNuggets	4 oz.	283	18	5 Grams	57%
McDonald's French Fries	3 oz.	222	12	5 Grams	49%
McDonald's Chocolate Shake	11 oz.	356	10	6 Grams	25%
Kentucky Fried Chicken (2 piece)	6 oz.	460	31	7 Grams	61%
Kentucky Fried Chicken Nuggets	4 oz.	281	17	4 Grams	54%

Food Product	Weight	Calories	Total Fat Grams	Saturated Fat	Fat Calories
Kentucky Fried Chicken French Fries	3 oz.	249	13	2 Grams	47%
Roy Roger's Roast Beef	6 oz.	335	11	3 Grams	30%
Roy Roger's Chicken (2 piece)	6 oz.	519	35	8 Grams	61%
Roy Roger's French Fries	3 oz.	237	13	4 Grams	49%
Roy Roger's Chocolate Shake	12 oz.	430	11	6 Grams	23%
Wendy's Big Classic	8 oz.	500	28	11 Grams	50%
Wendy's Chicken Filet Sandwich	8 oz.	479	24	7 Grams	45%
Wendy's French Fries	3 oz.	287	14	4 Grams	44%
Wendy's Chocolate Frosty	9 oz.	351	13	6 Grams	33%

Table 2

Menu Item	Weight	Calories	Total Fat Grams	Saturated Fat Grams	Fat Calories
Hamburgers					
Burger King Whopper	9 oz.	584	33	13	51%
McDonald's Big Mac	7 oz.	572	34	15	53%
Wendy's Big Classic	8 oz.	500	28	11	50%
Roast Beef					
Arby's (regular)	5 oz.	365	19	7	47%
Hardee's (regular)	5 oz.	338	17	6	45%
Roy Roger's	6 oz.	335	11	3	30%
Fish					
Burger King Whaler	6 oz.	478	26	3	49%
McDonald's Filet-O-Fish	5 oz.	415	23	5	50%
Chicken					
Arby's Chicken Breast Sandwich	7 oz.	567	32	7	51%
Burger King Chicken Tenders	3 oz.	223	12	3	48%

Menu Item	Weight	Calories	Total Fat Grams	Saturated Fat Grams	Fat Calories
Church's Fried Chicken 2 piece	6 oz.	487	35	9	65%
Hardee's Chicken Filet Sandwich	7 oz.	431	20	6	42%
Kentucky Fried Chicken 2 piece	6 oz.	460	31	7	61%
Kentucky Fried Chicken Nuggets	4 oz.	281	18	5	58%
Roy Roger's Chicken 2 piece	6 oz.	519	35	8	61%
Wendy's Chicken Sandwich	8 oz.	479	24	7	45%
French Fries					
Arby's	3 oz.	222	11	3	45%
Burger King	3 oz.	255	13	5	46%
Church's Fried Chicken	4 oz.	338	16	5	43%
Hardee's	3 oz.	230	12	4	47%
Kentucky Fried Chicken	3 oz.	249	13	2	47%
McDonald's	3 oz.	222	12	5	49%
Roy Rogers	3 oz.	237	13	4	49%
Wendy's	3 oz.	287	14	4	44%
Chocolate Shakes					
Arby's	11 oz.	426	14	7	30%
Burger King	11 oz.	351	10	5	26%
Hardee's	11 oz.	349	11	6	28%
McDonald's	11 oz.	356	10	6	25%
Roy Rogers	12 oz.	430	11	6	23%
Wendy's Frosty	9 oz.	351	13	6	33%

Fast Food Addresses

Arby's
Consumer Affairs,
 Arby's Inc.
Ten Piedmont Center, Suite 700
3495 Piedmont Road
Atlanta, Georgia 30305

Burger King
Consumer Information,
 Burger King Corporation
1777 Old Cutler Road
Miami, Florida 33157

Frisch's Big Boy Restaurant
 Incorporated
Consumer Affairs Office
2800 Gilbert Avenue
Cincinnati, Ohio 45206

Hardee's
Hardee Food Systems
P.O. Box 1619
Rocky Mount, North Carolina
27804-2805

Kentucky Fried Chicken
Public Affairs Department
KFC Corporation
P.O. Box 32070
Louisville, Kentucky 40232

McDonald's
McDonald's Nutrition
 Information Center
McDonald's Plaza
Oak Brook, Illinois 60521

Pizza Hut
Pizza Hut
 Information Center
P.O. Box 484
911 East Douglas
Wichita, Kansas 67202

RAX
RAX Restaurants
 Consumer Affairs
1317 East Broad Street
Columbus, Ohio 43205

Roy Rogers
Roy Rogers Division of
 Frisch's Big Boy Restaurants
Consumer Affairs Office
2800 Gilbert Avenue
Cincinnati, Ohio 45206

Wendy's
Consumer Affairs
 Department
Wendy's International, Inc.
P.O. Box 256
Dublin, Ohio 43017

For questions or additional information please write to us at:

Cardiovascular Education Specialists
P.O. Box 42346
Cincinnati, Ohio 45242

Be sure to include your question along with your name and address and we will answer questions or provide additional information to you.

Selected References

Chapter 1

American Heart Association. *1993 Heart & Stroke Facts.*

Lipid Research Clinics Program. (1984). The Lipid Research Clinics Coronary Primary Prevention Trial results: I. Reduction in the incidence of coronary heart disease. *Journal of the American Medical Association, 251,* 351–364.

Lipid Research Clinics Program. (1984). The Lipid Research Clinics Coronary Primary Prevention Trial results: II. The relationship of reduction in incidence of coronary heart disease to cholesterol lowering. *Journal of the American Medical Association, 251,* 365–374.

National Institutes of Health Consensus Conference Statement. (1984). Lowering blood cholesterol to prevent heart disease, Vol. 5, No. 7. U.S. Department of Health and Human Services, National Institutes of Health Office of Medical Applications of Research, Building 1, Room 216, Bethesda, Maryland 20205.

National Institutes of Health, National Cholesterol Education Program. (September 1993). Second report of the expert panel: Detection, evaluation, and treatment of high cholesterol in adults (Adult Treatment Panel II) NIH

Publication No. 93-3095, National Institutes of Health National Heart, Lung, and Blood Institute.

Stamler J., Wentworth D., Neaton J., and others. (1986). Is relationship between serum cholesterol and risk of premature death from coronary heart disease continuous or graded? *Journal of the American Medical Association, 256,* 2823–2828.

Chapter 2

American Academy of Pediatrics Committee on Nutrition. (1986). Prudent life-style for children: Dietary fat and cholesterol. *Pediatrics, 78,* 521–525.

Ginsburg, G. S. and Pasternak, R. C. (1994). How and when to lower lipid levels in patients with established CAD. *Journal of Critical Care Illness, 9* (11), 993–1024.

Gotto, A. M., Jr. (1990). Interrelationship of triglycerides with lipoproteins and high-density lipoproteins. *American Journal of Cardiology, 66* (6), 20A–23A.

Grundy, S. (1986). Cholesterol and coronary heart disease: A new era. *Journal of the American Medical Association, 256,* 2849–2858.

LaRosa, J. C. (1990). At what levels of total low- or high-density lipoprotein cholesterol should diet/drug therapy be initiated? *American Journal of Cardiology, 65,* (12), 7F–10F.

Mann, G. V. (1994). Metabolic consequences of dietary trans fatty acids. *The Lancet, 343* (8908), 1268–1271.

Report of the National Cholesterol Education Program Expert Panel on Detection, Evaluation, and Treatment of High Blood Cholesterol in Adults. (1988). *Archives Internal Medicine, 148,* 36–69.

Rudel, L., Parks, J., Johnson, F., Babiak, J. (1986). Low density lipoproteins in atherosclerosis. *Journal of Lipid Research, 27,* 465–474.

Slyper, A. H. (1994). Low-density lipoprotein density and atherosclerosis. *Journal of the American Medical Association,* 272 (4), 305–308.

Thuesen, L., Henriksen, L., Engby, B. (1986). One-year experience with a low-fat, low-cholesterol diet in patients with coronary heart disease. *The American Journal of Clinical Nutrition, 44,* 212–219.

U.S. Department of Health and Human Services, Public Health Service, National Institutes of Health. Cholesterol counts: steps to lowering your patient's blood cholesterol; cholesterol management principles from the coronary primary prevention trial. NIH Publication No. 85-2699.

Wynder, E., Field, F., Haley, N. (1986). Population screening for cholesterol determination: A pilot study. *Journal of the American Medical Association, 256,* 2839–2842.

Chapter 3

Austin, M. A. (1991). Plasma triglyceride and coronary artery disease. *Arteriosclerosis & Thrombosis, 11* (1), 2–14.

Austin, M. A., Hokanson, J. E. (1994). Epidemiology of triglycerides, small dense low-density lipoprotein, and lipoprotein (a) as risk factors for coronary heart disease. *Medical Clinics of North America, 78* (1), 99–115.

Geurian, K., Pinson, J. B., Weart, C. W. (1992). The triglyceride connection in atherosclerosis. *Annals of Pharmacotherapy, 26* (9), 1109–1117.

Gotto, A. M., Jr. (1992). Interrelationship of triglycerides with lipoproteins and high density lipoproteins. *American Journal of Cardiology, 66* (6), 20A–23A.

Pearson, T. A. (1992). Theraputic management of triglycerides: An international perspective. *American Journal of Cardiology, 70* (19), 26H–31H.

Steiner, G. (1993). Triglyceride-rich lipoproteins and atherosclerosis, from fast to feast. *Annals of Medicine, 25* (5), 431–435.

Chapter 4

Ballard-Barbash, R., Callaway, C. W. (1987). Marine fish oils: Role in prevention of coronary artery disease. *Mayo Clinic Proceedings, 62*, 113–118.

Becker, D., Brown Wilder, L., Pearson, T. (1986). Hypercholesterolemia: Nutritional and pharmacoligic management. *Maryland Medical Association Journal, 35*, 549–551.

Grundy, S. (1986). Comparison of monounsaturated fatty acids and carbohydrates for plasma cholesterol lowering. *New England Journal of Medicine, 314*, 745–748.

Keys, A. (1984). Serum cholesterol response to dietary cholesterol. *American Journal of Clinical Nutrition, 40*, 351–359.

Kinsella, J. (1986). Dietary fish oils. *Nutrition Today*, Nov.–Dec., 7–14.

Mattson, F., Grundy, S. (1985). Comparison of dietary saturated, monounsaturated, and polyunsaturated fatty acids on plasma lipids and lipoproteins in man. *Journal Lipid Research, 26*, 194–202.

Nutrition and the M.D. A continuing education service for physicians and nutritionists, 1986, 12.

U.S. Department of Health and Human Services, Public Health Service, National Institutes of Health. Facts about blood cholesterol. NIH Publication No. 85-2696.

Chapter 5

American Heart Association. An eating plan for healthy Americans. AHA publication 51-018-B(SA).

American Heart Association. (1986). Dietary guidelines for healthy American adults: A statement for physicians and health professionals by the Nutrition Committee, American Heart Association, 74, 1465A–1468A.

American Heart Association. Eating for a healthy heart: Dietary treatment of hyperlipidemia. AHA publication 50-063-A.

American Heart Association. The way to a man's heart. AHA publication 51-08-A.

Chang, N. W., Huang, P. C. (1990). Effects of dietary monounsaturated fatty acids on plasma lipids in humans. *Journal of Lipid Research, 31* (12), 2141–2147.

Consensus Development Conference. (1985). Lowering blood cholesterol to prevent heart disease. *Journal of the American Medical Assocation, 253,* 2080–2086.

Dreon, D. M., Vranizan, K. M., Krauss, R. M., Austin, M. A., Wood, P. D. (1990). The effect of polyunsaturated fat vs. monounsaturated fat on plasma lipoproteins. *Journal of the American Medical Assocation, 263* (18), 2462–2466.

Foley, M., Ball, M., Chisholm, A., Duncan, A., Spears, G., Mann, J. (1992). Should mono- or poly-unsaturated fats replace saturated fat in the diet? *European Journal of Clinical Nutrition, 46* (6), 429–436.

Ginsberg, H. N., Barr, S. L., Gilbert, A., Karmally, W., Deckelbaum, R., Kaplan, K., Ramakrishnan, R., Hollaran, S., Dell, R. B. (1990). Reduction of plasma cholesterol levels in normal men on an American Heart Association Step I or a Step II diet with added monounsaturated fat. *New England Journal of Medicine, 322* (9), 574–579.

Grundy, S., Bilheimer, D., Blackburn, H., and others. (1982). Rationale of the Diet Heart Statement of the American Heart Association: Report of Nutrition Committee, *Circulation, 65,* 839A–854A.

Lichtenstein, A. H., Ausman, L. M., Carrasco, W., Jenner, J. L., Gualtieri, L. J., Goldin, B. R., Ordovas, J. M., Schaefer, E. J. (1993). Effects of canola, corn, and olive oils on fasting and postprandial plasma lipoproteins in humans as part of a National Cholesterol Education Program Step II Diet. *Arteriosclerosis & Thrombosis, 13* (10), 1533–1542.

Mata, P., Alvarez-Sala, L. A., Rubio, M. J., Nuno, J., De Oya, M. (1992). Effects of long term monounsaturated vs. polyunsaturated enriched diets on lipoproteins in healthy men and women. *American Journal of Clinical Nutrition, 55* (4), 846–850.

Mensink, R. P., Katan, M. B. (1990). Effects of dietary trans fatty acids on high-density and low-density lipoprotein cholesterol levels in healthy subjects. *New England Journal of Medicine, 323* (7), 439–445.

U.S. Department of Health and Human Services, Public Health Service, National Institutes of Health: So you have high blood cholesterol . . .; NIH publication No. 87-2922.

Chapter 6

Lichtenstein, A. H., Ausman, L. M., Carrasco, W., Jenner, J. L., Ordovas, J. M., Schaefer, E. J. (1994). Hypercholesterolemic effect of dietary cholesterol in diets enriched in polyunsaturated and saturated fat. Dietary cholesterol, fat saturation, and plasma lipids. *Arteriosclerosis & Thrombosis, 14* (1) 168–175.

Chapter 7

Lowering Blood Cholesterol to Prevent Heart Disease. National Institutes of Health Consensus Development Conference Statement; Vol. 5, No. 7.

Report of the National Cholesterol Education Program Expert Panel on Detection, Evaluation, and Treatment of High Blood Cholesterol in Adults. (1988). *Archives of Internal Medicine, 148,* 36–69.

U. S. Department of Health and Human Services, Public Health Service, National Institutes of Health. Cholesterol management principles from the coronary primary prevention trial; NIH publication No. 85-2699.

U.S. Department of Health and Human Services, Public Health Service, National Institutes of Health. NIH publication No. 87-2920.

Chapter 8

Glueck, C. (1985). Drugs that affect high-density lipoprotein cholesterol levels: mechanisms of action and relationships to coronary heart disease. *Internal Medicine* 1985 special issue, 20–25.

Report of the National Cholesterol Education Program Expert Panel on Detection, Evaluation, and Treatment of High Blood Cholesterol in Adults. (1988). *Archives of Internal Medicine, 148,* 36–69.

Chapter 9

Anderson, K., Castelli, W., Levy, D. (1987). Cholesterol and mortality: 30 years of follow-up from the Framingham study. *Journal of the American Medical Association, 257,* 2176–2180.

Castelli, W. (1983). Cardiovascular disease and multifactorial risk: Challenge of the 1980s. *American Heart Journal, 106,* 1191–1200.

Clifton, P. M., Nestel, P. J. (1992). Influence of gender, body mass index, and age on response of plasma lipids to dietary fat plus cholesterol. *Arteriosclerosis & Thrombosis, 12* (8), 955–962.

Despres, J. P., Moorjani, S., Lupien, P. J., Tremblay, A., Nadeau, A., Bouchard, C. (1990). Regional distribution of body fat, plasma lipoproteins and cardiovascular disease. *Arteriosclerosis, 10* (4), 495–511.

Dwyer, J., and others. (1988). Low level cigarette smoking and longitudinal change in serum cholesterol among adolescents, the Berlin-Bremen study. *Journal of the American Medical Association, 259,* 2857–2862.

Kuczmarski, R. J., Flegal, K. M., Campbell, S. M., Johnson, C. L. (1994). Increasing prevalence of overweight among U.S. adults (the national health and nutrition surveys, 1960–1991). *Journal of the American Medical Association, 273* (3), 205–237.

Multiple Risk Factor Intervention Trial Research Group. (1982). Multiple risk factor intervention trial, risk factor changes and mortality results. *Journal of the American Medical Association, 248,* 1465–1477.

Multiple Risk Factor Intervention Trial Research Group. (1986). Coronary heart disease, death, nonfatal acute myocardial infarction and other clinical outcomes in the multiple risk factor intervention trial. *American Journal of Cardiology, 58*, 1–9.

Warwick, Z. S., Schiffman, S. S. (1992). Role of dietary fat in calorie intake and weight gain. *Neuroscience & Behavioral Reviews, 16* (4), 585-596.

Chapter 10
Berg, A., Frey, I., Baumstark, M. W., Halle, M., Keul, J. (1994). Physical activity and lipoprotein lipid disorders. *Sports Medicine, 17* (1), 6–21.

Johnson C., Greenland, P. (1990). Effects of exercise, dietary cholesterol, and dietary fat on blood lipids. *Archives of Internal Medicine, 150* (1), 137–141.

Krummel, D., Etherton, T. D., Peterson, S., Kris-Etherton, P. M. Effects of exercise on plasma lipids and lipoproteins of women. *Proceedings of the Society for Experimental Biology & Medicine, 204* (2), 123–137.

Pronk, N. P. (1993). Short term effects of exercise on plasma lipid and lipoproteins in humans. *Sports Medicine, 16* (6), 431–448.

Superko, H. R. (1991). Exercise training, serum lipids and lipoprotein particles: Is there a change threshold? *Medicine & Science in Sports & Exercise, 23* (6), 677–685.

Chapter 11
Hachey, D. L. (1994). Benefits and risks of modifying maternal fat intake in pregnancy and lactation. *American Journal of Clinical Nutrition, 59* (2 Suppl.), 454S–464S.

Kesteloot, H., Sasaki, S. (1993). On the relationship between nutrition, sex hormones and high-density lipoproteins in women. *ACTA Cardiologica, 48* (4), 355–363.

Knopp, R. H. (1990). Effects of sex hormones on lipoprotein levels in pre- and post-menopausal women. *Canadian Journal of Cardiology, 6* (Suppl. B), 31B–35B.

Krummel, D., Etherton, T. D., Peterson, S., Kris-Etherton, P. M. (1993). Effects of exercise on plasma lipids and lipoproteins of women. *Proceedings of the Society for Experimental Biology & Medicine, 204* (2), 123–137.

LaRosa, J. C. (1992). Women, lipoproteins and cardiovascular disease risk. *International Journal of Fertility, 37* (Suppl. 2), 63–71.

Chapter 12
Birch, L. L. (1992). Children's preferences for high fat foods. *Nutrition Reviews, 50* (9), 249–255.

Quivers, E. S., Driscoll, D. J., Garvey, C. D., Harris, A. M., Harrison, J., Huse, D. M., Murtaugh, P., Weidman, W. H. (1992). Variability in response to a low-fat cholesterol diet in children with elevated low-density lipoprotein cholesterol levels. *Pediatrics, 89* (5Pt.1), 925–929.

Thompson, F. E., Dennison, B. A. (1994). Dietary sources of fats and cholesterol in U.S. children aged 2 through 5 years. *American Journal of Public Health, 84* (5), 799–806.

Weidman, W. H. (1992). Variability in response to a low-fat cholesterol diet in children with elevated low-density lipoprotein cholesterol levels. *Pediatrics, 89* (5Pt.1), 925–929.

Whitaker, R. C., Wright, J. A., Finch, A. J., Deyo, R. A., Psaty, B. M. (1993). School lunch: A comparison of the fat and cholesterol content with dietary guidelines. *Journal of Pediatrics, 123* (6), 857–862.

Chapter 13
Coronary Drug Project Research Group. (1975). Colfibrate and niacin in coronary heart disease. *Journal of the American Medical Association, 231,* 360–381.

Helsinki Heart Study. (1987). Primary prevention trial with Gemfibrozil in middle-aged men with dyslipidemia. *New England Journal of Medicine, 317.*

Levey, R. I., Troendle, A. J., Fattu, J. M. (1993). A quarter century of drug treatment of dyslipoproteinemia, with a focus on the new HMG-CoA reductase inhibitor fluvastatin. *Circulation, 87* (4 Suppl.), III 45–53.

Lipid Research Clinics Coronary Primary Prevention Trial Results. (1984). I. Reduction in incidence of coronary disease. II. The relationship of reduction in incidence of coronary heart disease to cholesterol lowering. *Journal of the American Medical Association, 251,* 351–365.

Lovastatin Study Group. (1986). Therapeutic response to lovastatin (mevinolin) in nonfamilial hypercholesterolemia. *Journal of the American Medical Association, 256,* 2829–2834.

Scandinavian Simvastatin Survival Study Group: Randomized trial of cholesterol lowering in 4444 patients with coronary heart disease. (1994). The Scandinavian Simvastatin Survival Study (4S). *The Lancet, 344,* 1383–1389.

Schaefer, E.J. (1994). Familial lipoprotein disorders and premature coronary artery disease. *Medical Clinics of North America, 78* (1), 21–39.

Shepherd, J., and others. (1979). The effects of cholestyramine on high-density lipoprotein metabolism. *Atherosclerosis, 33,* 433.

Sheperd, J., and others. (1979). Effects of nicotinic acid therapy on plasma high-density lipoprotein subfraction distribution and composition and on appoliprotein A metabolism. *Journal of Clinical Investigation, 63,* 858–862.

Smith, H. T., Jokubaitis, L. A., Troendle, A. J., Hwang, D. S., Robinson, W. T. (1993). Pharmacokinetics of Fluvastatin and specific drug interactions. *American Journal of Hypertension,* 6 (11 Pt.2), 375–382.

Vega, G., Grundy, S. (1987). Treatment of primary moderate hypercholesterolemia with lovastatin (mevinolin) and Colestipol. *Journal of the American Medical Association, 257,* 33–38.

Chapter 14
American Heart Association. Dining Out: A guide to restaurant dining. AHA publication 50-067(CP).

Chapter 15

Masser, P. A., Taylor, L. M., Porter, J. M. (1994). Importance of elevated plasma homocysteine levels as a risk factor for atherosclerosis. *Annals of Thorasic Surgery, 58,* 1240–1246.

Meydani, M. (1992). Vitamin E requirement in relation to dietary fish oil and oxidative stress in elderly. *EXS, 62,* 411–418.

Meyers, D. G., Maloley, P. A. (1993). The antioxidant vitamins: impact on atherosclerosis. *Pharmacotherapy, 13* (6), 574–582.

Chapter 16

American Heart Association. Recipes for fat-controlled, low-cholesterol meals. AHA publication 50-020(CP).

The American Heart Association Cookbook, 4th ed., M. Winston, R. Eshleman, 1984. David McKay Co., New York.

Diet for a Healthy Heart. (1985). Fleischmann's for Nabisco Brands, Inc.

Glossary

Adenosine triphosphate (ATP)   The high-energy phosphate molecule that provides energy for cellular function.

Aerobic exercise   A method of exercise that conditions the cardiovascular system by using movements that create an increased demand for oxygen over an extended period of time.

Angina pectoris   A reversible condition in which the heart muscle temporarily does not receive a sufficient supply of blood. This decreased blood supply to the heart occurs when the coronary arteries are blocked with cholesterol and fatty deposits, limiting the flow of blood that is necessary for the heart to function properly. When restricted blood flow to the heart occurs, the person may experience discomfort. Most typically this discomfort occurs in the chest, but it may be in the arms, shoulders, neck, or back. The discomfort is most often described as pain, pressure, burning, or squeezing.

Antioxidants   Some vitamins, such as E and beta carotene, which possess antioxidant properties. Since oxidation is one of the first steps in producing atherosclerosis, it has been postulated that vitamins with antioxidant properties may help prevent heart disease.

Atherosclerosis   This condition is commonly called "hardening of the arteries." It is a progressive disease that causes the arteries to narrow and the walls of the arteries to lose their elasticity. The arteries are narrowed and hardened when cholesterol and fats build up in the walls of the arteries. When atherosclerosis occurs in the coronary arteries, the heart muscle does not receive the blood and nutrients it needs, and this leads to angina pectoris and possibly a heart attack.

Bile acid sequestrants   A group of medications used to treat abnormally high blood cholesterol levels. The bile acid sequestrants bind the cholesterol contained in the bile acids in the intestine. When the cholesterol has been bound by the bile acid sequestrant, it is eliminated from the body in the stool.

Blood cholesterol   All cholesterol that is found in the blood. Blood cholesterol is the cholesterol that the body manufactures in addition to the exogenous cholesterol from dietary fats and cholesterol. Blood cholesterol is one of the factors in the development of atherosclerosis.

Cholesterol   A fatty substance that is necessary for many bodily functions. It is endogenously produced by the human body and by all animals, including fish and fowl.

Coronary arteries   The blood vessels that carry blood rich in oxygen and nutrients to the heart. When the coronary arteries become narrowed with atherosclerosis, angina pectoris and heart attack can occur. Any disease of the coronary artery is referred to as coronary artery disease.

Diabetes   A chronic disease that affects the body's use of carbohydrates and fats. People with diabetes often have abnormal blood cholesterol levels.

Dietary cholesterol   Cholesterol that is found in the foods you eat. Dietary cholesterol is found only in food from animal sources. Dietary cholesterol contributes to the elevation of blood cholesterol and the subsequent development of atherosclerosis.

Diuretic   A medication that is used to increase the production of urine. Frequently referred to as a water pill, diuretics may be used to control hypertension. Some diuretics may increase total blood cholesterol.

Fat   One of three types of nutrients that supply energy to the body. Fats contain nine calories in every gram. Fats are found in three different types: saturated, polyunsaturated, and monounsaturated.

Heart attack   Irreversible damage to the heart muscle that results from a decreased or lack of blood supply to the heart muscle. This is frequently caused by atherosclerosis.

Heart disease   Any disease of the heart, including diseases of the muscle, coronary arteries, and valves. The most common type of heart disease is that caused by atherosclerosis, leading to angina pectoris and heart attack.

High density lipoprotein (HDL)   This is the portion of the blood lipids that removes cholesterol deposits and low density lipoproteins (LDL) from the blood. HDL carries cholesterol and LDL to the liver, where it is broken down and excreted from the body. HDL is the "good" fraction of cholesterol. It is desirable to have a high HDL cholesterol in the blood.

HMG CoA reductase Inhibitors   A type of medication used to lower blood cholesterol levels. This family of medications blocks the production of cholesterol in the liver by stopping the action of a necessary enzyme. When the liver is prohibited from making cholesterol, absorption of cholesterol from the blood is increased to meet the body's demands. The liver increases its absorption of cholesterol from the blood by increasing the number of places that LDL cholesterol can be received into the liver. Since the liver is removing LDL cholesterol from the blood, there is less LDL cholesterol left in the blood. In various studies, the family of HMG CoA reductase Inhibitors reduces blood LDL cholesterol and total cholesterol. In addition, triglycerides may decrease, and HDL cholesterol has a tendency to increase.

Hydrogenation   A process that converts liquid vegetable oil into a more solid product. The more an oil is hydrogenated, the more saturated fat it contains.

Hypercholesterolemia An elevation in the cholesterol level found in the blood.

Hypertension High blood pressure.

Lactic acid A product that results from the anaerobic metabolism of sugars, known to cause localized muscle fatigue and soreness.

Lipid Any fatty substance that is found in the body. The classification lipid includes cholesterol and triglycerides. Lipids are found in both blood and tissue in the body.

Lipoprotein Lipids that are combined with protein for transport through the blood. Lipoproteins are categorized by their density; LDL are low-density lipoproteins and HDL are high-density lipoproteins.

Low density lipoprotein (LDL) The largest amount of cholesterol is found in low density lipoproteins. LDL is deposited in the walls of arteries and is associated with atherosclerosis. LDL is referred to as "bad" cholesterol.

Monounsaturated fat One type of fat that is available in foods. Monounsaturated fats have been shown to lower total cholesterol by lowering the "bad" LDL. Olive, canola (rapeseed), and peanut oil are all monounsaturated fats.

Obesity The excess accumulation and storage of body fat. Typically defined as at least 20% above ideal body weight, or more than 30% body fat for women and more than 23% body fat for men.

Overweight A term to describe an excessive amount of weight for any given height.

Polyunsaturated fat A type of fat that is found in foods of plant or vegetable origin. Polyunsaturated fats have been found to lower total cholesterol. However, they do this by lowering both the LDL (bad) cholesterol as well as the HDL (good) cholesterol.

Risk factor A condition that is associated with an increased risk of developing heart disease. These conditions may be genetic traits, habits, or conditions. Some risk factors are elevated blood cholesterol, hypertension, smoking, male gender, family history, diabetes, obesity, sedentary lifestyle, and increased stress.

Saturated fat   A fat that is found primarily in foods of animal origin. Saturated fats are also found in palm and coconut. Saturated fats elevate the blood cholesterol more than any other dietary influence. To help reduce the risk of heart disease, saturated fat should be limited. Recommendations are to limit the total saturated fat to less than 10% of the total daily calorie intake.

Super obesity   Accumulation and storage of an excessive amount of body fat. Usually defined as 30% above the ideal body weight.

Triglycerides   A type of lipid found on the blood and tissue of humans and animals. Most of the body's fat stores are triglycerides. Elevated triglycerides are associated with an increased incidence of heart disease.

Unsaturated fat   Monounsaturated and polyunsaturated fats are types of unsaturated fat. The intake of monounsaturated and polyunsaturated fats should be limited to help reduce the risk of elevated cholesterol and consequently heart disease. Monounsaturated fats should be limited to less than 15% of total daily calorie intake. Polyunsaturated fat should be limited to about 7% or less than 10% of the total daily calorie intake.

Index

A

Adipose (fat) cells, storage of dietary fats in, 9

Alcohol
calories in, 132–33
consumption of, triglyceride levels lowered by decreasing, 12, 133

American diet as high in cholesterol and saturated fats, 8, 56, 65

American Heart Association (AHA)
blood cholesterol level recommended by, 56–57
deaths from voluntary cigarette smoking reported by, 88
dietary recommendations of, 23–24, 26–27, 103
recommendations for lowering cholesterol of, 75
restaurants and airlines that use food guidelines of, 123
statistics about annual heart attack rates of, 1
Step I and Step II diets of. *See* Step I diet and Step II diet
view of EDTA chelation therapy of, 142

Anabolic steroids, blood cholesterol levels raised by, 66

Aneurysm, atherosclerosis leading to, 1

Animal products
as high in cholesterol, 86
as high in saturated fats, 14, 152
vegetable sources as lower cholesterol choices than, 34

Antioxidants to stop oxidation of cholesterol, 141

Appetite defined, 80–81

Appetizers, selecting healthful, 128

"Apple" body type, 78

Atherosclerosis
accelerated by unsupervised administration of anabolic steroids, 66
defined, 3
EDTA chelation therapy to treat, 142
elevated blood cholesterol as causing, 1, 13
elevated triglyceride levels correlated with increased incidence of, 6
hardened buildup of cholesterol, fat, and calcium in, 3–4
lipids (HDL) that help to prevent, 6
lipids (LDL) that cause, 5–6, 99–100

Coconut oil
in breading, 149
as high in saturated fat, 14–16,
34, 128, 152
in ice milks and frozen
yogurt, 151
in nondairy toppings, 131
Coffee creamers
no-fat, 34
watching for coconut and
palm oils in, 15–16
Colestid
profile of, 118
to reduce cholesterol, 104–5
Colestipol HCl granules
profile of, 118
to reduce cholesterol, 104–5
Cooking tips for lowering
saturated fat and
cholesterol, 147–67
Cooking with fats and oils,
152–55
Cool-downs as beneficial to
body's systems, 73
Corn oil
low saturated fat in, 15
as polyunsaturated vegetable
fat, 17
Coronary artery disease. *See*
Coronary heart disease
(CHD)
Coronary heart disease
(CHD)
diabetes as risk factor for, 67
elevated blood cholesterol
levels as cause of, 1–2
low HDL and high LDL
cholesterol levels as risk
factors for, 91–92
recommended blood
cholesterol levels based
on levels of risk of
developing, 8
risks particular to women of,
92–95

role of triglycerides in,
10–11, 59
secondary prevention of high
blood cholesterol in adults
with evidence of, 116–17
sedentary lifestyle as risk
factor of, 71
study proving that lowering
blood cholesterol levels
reduces risk of, 2
Cottage cheese
no-fat, 34
substitution for, 53
Cottonseed oil as
polyunsaturated vegetable
fat, 17
Cream
in French cuisine, 138–39
in liquors, 133
saturated fats and cholesterol
in, 14
Cream cheese, no-fat, 34
Cream sauce, saturated fat in,
138, 152
Creamy yogurt chicken
alternative recipe, 162
Creamy yogurt sauce alternative
recipe, 163
Crispy southern chicken
alternative recipe, 159

D
Daily Cholesterol and Fat
Allowance Worksheet
blank, 31
examples of using, 27–29
instructions for calculations
on, 29–30
Daily fat calorie intake,
calculating, 25–31
Dairy products
to avoid, list of, 151–52
as high in saturated fats,
14, 34